HIV/AIDS MITIGATION

Policies, Programmes and Strategies in Manipur

About the Author

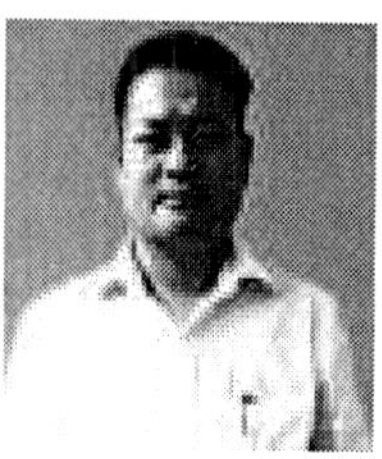

Dr. Lalzo S. Thangjom is currently working as Assistant Professor in the Department of Social Work, Assam (Central) University, Silchar , Assam. He obtained his Post-graduate degree in Social Work from Delhi University and Ph.D. Degree from Assam (Central) University Silchar, Assam. He received U G C Junior Research Fellowship award in December 2006. He has 14 years of teaching experience. His area of Acadmic interest includes Developmental Issues, Government and Politics, livelihood, Health Care, Inclusion and exclusion and community development. Substance Abuse and Deaddiction. Currently he is guiding Ph.D Scholars. He has contributed six chapters in edited books on Social Work Theory and Practice, Knowledge and Application and has written extensively on HIV and AIDS, the role of women, Issues of livelihood, entrepreneurial challenges, empowerment of tribal women and cultural identity in National and International Journal of repute.

HIV/AIDS Mitigation

Policies, Programmes and Strategies in Manipur

LALZO S. THANGJOM

Akansha Publishing House
Delhi • Guwahati • Visakhapatnam

AKANSHA PUBLISHING HOUSE
4649/21-B, Ansari Road
Daryaganj, New Delhi - 110 002
Phones: 23263193, 9435116718
Email: ektabooks@yahoo.com
Visit us: www.akanshapublishinghouse.com

HIV/AIDS Mitigation: ***Policies, Programmes and Strategies in Manipur***

First Published, 2021

ISBN 978-81-8370-596-7

PRINTED IN INDIA

Published by Akansha Publishing House, New Delhi - 110 002

Preface

It's been more than 50 years since the first case of HIV was detected in the western countries, nevertheless scientist and experts are still trying to find a cure for it. The best bet an HIV has is to attack the human immune system and then weakened it. Once the body's immune system is compromised, a host of Illness start knocking the human door. Cluster Division 4 in the red blood cell, which act as an antigen for illness is being attacked by HIV Virus and weakened their strength to protect human body.

It is with immense gratitude that I express my heartfelt thanks to my supervisor Dr. M. Tineshowri Devi, Professor, Department of Social Work, Assam University Silchar. Not only has she shown me the direction, but she has also helped in instilling into me a professional approach towards social issues and an attitude towards scientific research. Her guidance, concern, perseverance and, above all patience, are rare to come across. I thank her for the special measures she has taken in critical moments and motivated me to carry on the work.

My sincere thanks to various institution, libraries and documentation centre. Main among them are Delhi school of social work library, NCERT library New Delhi, Jamia Millia Islamia central and department of social work library, Manipur University central library, Assam University Central library and department of social work library Assam University. I am grateful to all the librarians and technical staff for extending a helping hand.

My colleagues and Head of Department Prof Subhabrata Dutta, Dr. Tarun Bikash Sukai, Dr. G. Albin Joseph, Dr. M. Gangabhusan, Mritunjay Singh, Dr. Kathiresan L. Dr. Kaivalya Desai and Mr. Ajit Kumar Jena deserves special thanks for their constant inputs and moral back up which motivates me always.

I express my sincere thanks to the staff of Manipur chief minister secretariat for their quick response in forwarding my application for data collection to the then health commissioner Shri Vumlunmang I.A.S and Manipur State AIDS Control Societies. I am also thankful to those entire organisation and specially their beneficiaries for giving me their valuable time in answering few of my questions. I express my thanks to all those politicians I have interviewed and technical staff of Manipur Assembly Secretariat.

My deepest gratitude to my maternal uncle Shri Lama B. Gangte for taking pain in translating assembly debates proceedings from Manipuri to English. Lastly I thank my family specially my Dad, Mom, Brothers, Sisters, my wife and my kids for their patience and understanding which have been a constant source of inspiration and support.

My debt of gratitude is acknowledged not only to those who have been mentioned, but also to those whose names have been inadvertently missed. It is their help and cooperation which has enabled me to achieve what I could.

Lalzo S. Thangjom

Contents

CHAPTER 1

Introduction

MANIPUR PROFILE

Manipur is a small state with a population of only 27.21 lakhs (2011 Census) and a land area of 22,327 sq. km. having an international boundary of 358 Km. with Myanmar. Manipur with hardly 0.2% of India's population is contributing nearly 8% of India's total HIV positive cases. Manipur being the border state to Myanmar which comes under the notorious golden triangle having a long history of Psychotropic substance use with opium and cannabis and pharmaceutical drugs use such as Buprenorphine or a cocktail with Antihistamine injections or sedative injection preparations like the Benzodiazepines coupled with sharing of contaminated syringes and needles, unsafe sexual practices under the influence of drugs is one of the most important factors making Injectible Drug Users (IDU) as major sources of infection. Trapped in an insurgent-affected zone together with the poor health delivery systems, Manipur needs to perceive the epidemic as an impending disaster of colossal proportion. Manipuri people and society are apparently sitting close to the volcano. In fact, there is growing realisation that there indeed is an association between insurgency, high drug use and HIV/AIDS.

There is a lingering political conflict and HIV/AIDS in the North Eastern states of India especially in Manipur. For the ordinary people and communities living in this area every new day comes up with fresh agenda for survival negotiations. Coping and management of fear is the most important concern cutting across class region in this area. In a scenario where even the press has its mouths regulated by the might of the barrel, or where every scheme and sanction has to first pass through the filter of the revolutionary groups. It's about time the civil societies roll up its sleeves and show genuine concern for real issues. "Governments in most conflict-affected Zones are not responding adequately to the threat of HIV/AIDS, for want of commitment and capacity building". (Subramanian K. S, 2002)

Despite each political party having HIV/AIDS Mitigations as their political Manifestoes, they are pressed with more immediate security and political concern and have no time for the HIV/AIDS causes. HIV/AIDS how it has affected the political economy and overall development of the state, in spite of the common belief that insurgency as the sole bottlenecks to economic development. The number of young people, who are infected, is increasing day by day. In Manipuri society, AIDS is becoming a disease of the young people (MSACS).

HIV/AIDS AND ITS REALITY

HIV/AIDS Stages, Modes of transmission and Prevention

The Acquired Immunodeficiency syndrome (AIDS) pandemic has become part of the contemporary global problems after its detection in the latter half of the 20th century. It is affecting the individual psycho-socio and political economy of all countries. Since the beginning of the pandemic, case definitions for Acquired Immunodeficiency Syndrome (AIDS) have undergone several revisions to respond to diagnostic and therapeutic advances and to improve standardization and comparability of surveillance data regarding persons at all stages of HIV disease.

The pandemic as it is defined by the American Centre for Disease Control (CDC); it is the presence of one of the 32 conditions indicative of severe immune-suppression associated with AIDS infection in an adult or adolescent aged 13 years or older.

Professionals from all fields have joined hands as it hardly needs to be mentioned that the AIDS has transcended geographical, socio-economic and political boundaries to find a solution to the challenge of the present century. Varying degrees of research by Medical, Social and Pharmaceuticals has been conducted but till date there has not been a real solution to halt the pandemic.

The Human Immunodeficiency Virus (HIV)

A Virus is a small organism which cannot be seen through our naked eyes but through a powerful microscope. Unlike other germs, a virus can reproduce itself only through entering a living cell and replacing or taking over some of the cell materials

White blood cells called macrophages and lymphocytes play an important role in the Human Immunodeficiency Virus (HIV) infection. When HIV enters the body, it binds itself to the lymphocytes, a type of white cells also called "helper cells" because they "instruct" other cells to fight off "foreign" intruders such as germs. HIV can enter T4 cells because they have what is called a CD4 receptor which matches the virus' key. Once HIV has entered these cells, its genetic material, RNA (Ribonucleic Acid), must be changed to match the cells' DNA (Deoxyribonucleic Acid). This is achieved with the help of enzymes. The invaded cells then begin to reproduce the virus, making hundreds of copies of HIV bursting out of their cells into the blood and lymph of their carrier host. T4 cells die about 24 to 36 hours after being infected with HIV. Although the body is able to replace them, their numbers decrease over time. As these cells are key agents in the immune response to various infections, their depletion eventually causes a serious deficit in normal antibodies, thereby opening the host body to all kinds of opportunistic infection infections.

Stages of HIV infection

Window period

This period refers to the time between the first exposure to HIV and "Seroconversion" that is the production of antibodies by the immune system in response to HIV infection. The person will not show any signs or symptoms at this point. The test result will be effective only after six week to six months from the initial contact.

Asymptomatic period

This is a period where HIV has already entered the human body and might already be there for several years. HIV works slowly and silently at this stage but started to destroy the T4 Cells. However there are no obvious signs and symptoms for the moment.

Symptomatic period

The host immune system is weakened by the killer virus at this stage and several of the HIV symptoms started to develop. Some of the most common symptoms include Diarrhoea, fever, drenching night sweats, persistent tiredness and several infections.

The stage of Acquired Immunodeficiency Syndrome

This is the last stages in HIV infection. Person living with HIV at this stage has a serious damage in the body Immune System. When a person is at this stage it would be marked by the emergence of several opportunistic infections like STI/STD's. All this infections are not directly caused by HIV but due to the consequences of HIV weakening the body immune system, thereby paving the way for other germs, bacteria and viruses.

Modes of HIV transmission

HIV can be transmitted from an infected person to someone else when there is an exchange of blood, semen or vaginal secretions. In addition, a baby born to an HIV-positive mother has a 14 to 25 per cent chance of being infected (The College of Family Physicians of Canada, 1995:23).

The Main modes of HIV transmissions are unprotected sexual intercourse with an infected partner, Injection or transfusion of contaminated blood or blood products, sharing of contaminated and unsterilized injecting equipment can also infect the other, Mother to child transmission (during pregnancy, at birth, and through breastfeeding), Occupational infections of healthcare or laboratory workers from contaminated needles pricking their bodies and came into contact with their blood also can infect them

Unprotected Sexual intercourse

Unprotected sexual intercourse with an infected partner was the most common form of infection during the past few years according to UNAIDS reports. Although receptive anal sex is estimated to produce the highest risk of infection, infection after a single insertive contact has also been described. The presence of other sexually transmitted infections also increases the risk of becoming infected with HIV.

Sharing of Contaminated Needles & Syringes

Sharing of unsterilized injecting equipment that has been previously used by someone who is infected is an important route of HIV transmission in many countries with a high prevalence of intravenous drug users. In contrast to the accidental needle stick injury, the risk of transmission through sharing injection equipment is far higher. According to Bradley M., et al 2008 in a study on Global epidemiology of injecting drug use and HIV among people who inject drugs says that Original TextInjecting drug use is an increasingly important cause of HIV transmission in most countries worldwide.

Mother to child transmission

An HIV infected mother can transmit infection to child during pregnancy and delivery in 15-30% of cases. In 75% of the cases the transmission is during delivery. In India, several thousand HIV-infected babies are born every year. Despite effective intervention, the identification of HIV infected pregnant women prior to delivery is a major problem. According to study conducted by Athena P. K., et al. (2006) concludes that for non-breastfeeding populations, 50% of HIV infections are transmitted to the infant at the very end of pregnancy, near to the time of labor. Also they add that transmission of the infection to the infant through breastfeeding is one of the main challenges in fighting paediatric HIV/AIDS in the developing world.

Contaminated blood transfusion

HIV can be transmitted through contaminated blood transfusion. Some people have been infected through a transfusion of infected blood. These days, all the blood used for transfusions in high-income countries is tested for HIV and HIV infection though infection through blood transfusions is now extremely rare. Yet this is not the case in some middle- and low-income countries, where there is lack of adequate blood safety procedures and measures are in place.

Prevention of HIV transmission

For each route of transmission there are things that an individual can do to reduce or eliminate risk. According to Mayer K and Pizer H, 2009 there are also interventions that have been proven to work at the community, local and national level. Wherever there is HIV, all three routes of transmission will take place. However the number of infections resulting from each route will vary greatly between countries and population groups. The share of resources allocated to each area should reflect the nature of the local epidemic - for example, if most infections occur among men who have sex with men then this group should be a primary target for prevention efforts.

According to *UNAIDS guidelines for HIV prevention 2007* "Knowing the epidemic in a particular region or country is the first, essential step in identifying, selecting and funding the most appropriate and effective HIV prevention measures for that country or region." -

HIV prevention should be comprehensive, making use of all approaches known to be effective rather than just implementing one or a few select actions in isolation. Successful HIV prevention program not only give information, but also build skills and provide access to essential commodities such as condoms or sterile injecting equipment. It should be remembered that many people don't fit into only one "risk category". For example, injecting drug users need access to condoms and safer sex counseling as well as support to reduce the risk of transmission through blood.

HIV prevention needs to reach both people who are at risk of HIV infection and those who are already infected: People who do not have HIV need interventions that will enable them to protect themselves from becoming infected. According to Kalichman S. (ed) (2006) People who are already living with HIV need knowledge and support to protect their own health and to ensure that they don't transmit HIV to others - known as "positive prevention". Positive prevention has become increasingly important as improvements in treatment have led to a rise in the number of people living with HIV.

According to Richardson et al (2004), counseling and testing are fundamental for HIV prevention. People living with HIV are less likely to transmit the virus to others if they know they are infected and if they have received counselling about safer behaviour. For example, a pregnant woman who has HIV will not be able to benefit from interventions to protect her child unless her infection is diagnosed. Those who discover they are not infected can also benefit, by receiving counselling on how to remain uninfected.

The availability and accessibility of antiretroviral treatment is crucial; it enables people living with HIV to enjoy longer, healthier lives, and as such acts as an incentive for HIV testing. Continued contact with health care workers also provides further opportunities for prevention messages and interventions. According to founding by Kennedy et al (2007) suggest that HIV-positive people may be less likely to engage in risky behaviour if they are enrolled in treatment programmes.

Prevention of HIV from contaminated blood transfusion

It is a well known fact that HIV is transmitted through contaminated blood and blood products. Government and medical professional have strived hard to limit the virus from infecting more and more people through this channel. In India during the later part of the 20th century the Supreme Court has banned professional blood donors from donating blood. Also, the government through its various hospitals and blood banks has taken up a stringent measure to ensure that safe blood is available through the blood banks. Transfusion of infected blood or blood products is the most efficient of all ways to transmit HIV. However, the chances of this happening can be greatly reduced by screening all blood supplies for the virus, and by heat-treating blood products where possible. In addition, because screening is not quite 100% accurate, it is sensible to place some restrictions on who is eligible to donate, provided that these are justified by epidemiological evidence, and don't unnecessarily limit supply or fuel prejudice. As UNAIDS, (1997) and WHO (2002) pointed out that reducing the number of unnecessary transfusions also helps to minimize risk. The safety of medical procedures and other activities that involve contact with blood, such as tattooing and circumcision, can be improved by routinely sterilizing equipment. An even better option is to dispose of equipment after each use, and this is highly recommended if at all possible.

Health care workers themselves run a risk of HIV infection through contact with infected blood. The most effective way for staff to limit this risk is to practice universal precautions, which means acting as though every patient is potentially infected. Universal precautions include washing hands and using protective barriers for direct contact with blood and other body fluids. (WHO Universal precautionary guidelines) Many resource-poor countries lack facilities for rigorously screening blood supplies. Takei T et al (2009) In addition a lot of countries have difficulty recruiting enough donors, and so have to resort to importing blood or paying their citizens to donate, which is not the best way to ensure safety.

Prevention of HIV from Contaminated Needles and Syringes

People, who share equipment to inject recreational drugs, have a very high risk of becoming infected with HIV from other drug users who have an HIV. Needle exchange programs have been shown to reduce the number of new HIV infections without encouraging drug use. These programs distribute clean needles and safely dispose off used ones, and also offer related services such as referrals to drug treatment centre's and HIV counseling and testing. According to WHO (2005) Needle exchanges are a necessary part of HIV prevention in any community that contains injecting drug users. Report made by WHO April (2004) also highlights the importance of community outreach for injecting drug users, small group counselling and other activities that encourage safer behaviour and access to available prevention options.

Despite the evidence that they do not encourage drug use, some authorities still refuse to support needle exchanges and other programs to help injecting drug users. Restrictions on pharmacies selling syringes without prescriptions, and on possession of drug paraphernalia, can also hamper HIV prevention programs by making it harder for drug users to avoid sharing equipment.

In much of the world the safety of medical procedures in general is compromised by lack of resources, and this may put both patients and staff at greater risk of HIV infection.

Prevention of HIV through Sexual Transmission

One can prevent HIV through sexual transmission by following these guidelines: Abstaining from sex, being faithful to one partner, using of male or female condoms consistently and correctly

Studies conducted by Lamptey and Price (1998) shows that there are a number of effective ways to encourage people to adopt safer sexual behavior, including media campaigns, social marketing, peer education and small group counseling. These activities should be carefully tailored to the needs and circumstances of the people they intend to help.

Findings by UNAIDS (2004) have shown that condoms, if used consistently and correctly, are highly effective at preventing HIV infection. Also there is no evidence that promoting condoms lead to increased sexual activity among young people. Therefore condoms should be made readily and consistently available to all those who need them.

However findings of Marston and King (2006) tell us that it is not easy for people to sustain changes in sexual behavior. In particular, young people often have difficulty remaining abstinent, and women in male-dominated societies are frequently unable to negotiate condom use, let alone abstinence. Many couples are compelled to have unprotected sex in order to have children. Other's associates condoms with promiscuity or lack of trust.

Prevention from Mother-to-child transmission

There are a number of things that can be done to help a pregnant woman with HIV to avoid passing her infection to her child. A course of antiretroviral drugs given to her during pregnancy and labor as well as to her newborn baby can greatly reduce the chances of the child becoming infected. Although the most effective treatment involves a combination of drugs taken over a long period, even a single dose of treatment can cut the transmission rate by half. Medical professionals also claim that a caesarean operation to deliver a baby through its mother's abdominal wall reduces the baby's exposure to its mother's body fluids and it lowers the risk of HIV transmission, but is likely to be recommended only if the mother has a high level of HIV in her blood, and if the benefit to her baby outweighs the risk of the intervention.

In much of the world a lack of drugs and medical facilities limits what can be done to prevent mother-to-child transmission of HIV. Antiretroviral drugs are not widely available in many resource-poor countries, caesarean section is often impractical, and many women lack the resources needed to avoid breastfeeding their babies. HIV/AIDS transmission from infected mother to child can be prevented by simple interventions such as antiretroviral transmission prophylaxis and elective caesarean section. This is also called the vertical transmission and in 10% of the time it can occur during the third trimester of pregnancy and another 10-15% of the time during breast feeding. This knowledge and understanding gives us an opportunity to prevent the spread from mother to child. It requires creating awareness among pregnant mothers to be treated themselves and approach hospitals which offer caesarean section for HIV infected women. HIV-related stigma is another obstacle in the prevention of mother-to-child transmission. Some women are afraid to attend clinics that distribute antiretroviral drugs, or to feed their babies formula, in case by doing so they reveal their HIV status.

EPIDEMIOLOGY GLOBAL AND INDIA

According to UNAIDS 2020, the total number of people living with HIV in 2019 is 38 million. Sub Saharan Africa continues to be ranked one with more than 20.7 Million HIV Positive followed

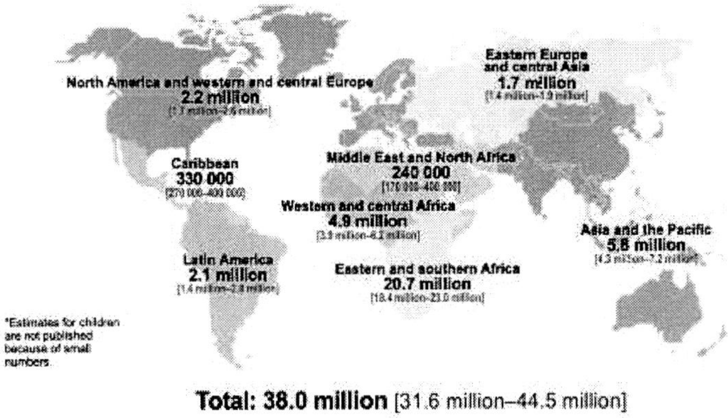
North America and western and central Europe
2.2 million
Eastern Europe and central Asia
1.7 million
Caribbean
330 000
Middle East and North Africa
240 000
Western and central Africa
4.9 million
Asia and the Pacific
5.8 million
Latin America
2.1 million
Eastern and southern Africa
20.7 million
*Estimates for children are not published because of small numbers.
Total: 38.0 million [31.6 million–44.5 million]

Picture: Global Adults and Children Living with HIV
Source: UNAIDS Global epidemiology update 2020

by Asia. North America and western and central Europe accounts for 2.2 million HIV Positive, Eastern Europe and Asia accounts for 1.7 Million

Asia is home to 60% of the world's population with diverse cultures and tradition ranked second only to sub-Saharan Africa in terms of the number of people living with HIV. According to estimates by UNAIDS India accounts for roughly half of Asia's HIV prevalence. With the exception of Thailand, every country in Asia has an adult HIV prevalence of less than 1%. Though Asia has a very large population, the low rate of HIV prevalence translates into a substantial portion of the global HIV burden. Though the rate of HIV prevalence might be low, it cannot escape the epidemic's harmful consequences.

Asia's epidemic has long been concentrated in specific populations, namely injecting drug users, men who have sex with men, sex workers and their clients. However, the epidemic in many parts of Asia is steadily expanding into lower-risk populations through transmission to the sexual partners of those most at risk.

HIV epidemic in India is concentrated among High Risk Groups and is heterogeneous in its distribution. The vulnerabilities that drive the epidemic are different in different parts of the country. Overall trends of HIV portray a declining epidemic at national level, though regional variations exist. The Department of AIDS Control has been monitoring levels and trends of HIV among different population groups to craft effective responses to control HIV/AIDS in India through the HIV Sentinel Surveillance System since 1998.

PUBLIC ISSUE (GLOBAL ASPECT)

The HIV since its detection in 1981 in the United States of America, it continues to baffle professionals from different fields. One by one it has engulfed populations in all countries of the world. HIV and AIDS have been widely recognized as the single greatest threat to sustainable development. For example, in sub-Saharan African countries, it has increased infant mortality and reduced life expectancy to levels not seen since the 1960s. Moreover, infant and child mortality rates are expected to double and even triple early in the next century. HIV/AIDS is a global problem requiring a global solution. It does not recognize boundaries of nationality, gender, age, occupation or sexual preference.

In spite of recent advances in treatment and care available in most developed countries, the HIV/AIDS pandemic continues to spread throughout the developing world. Structural inequalities continue to fuel the epidemic in all societies, and HIV infection has increasingly been concentrated in the poorest, most marginalized sectors of society in all countries. The relationship between HIV/AIDS and social and economic development has therefore become a central point in policy discussions about the most effective responses to the epidemic.

DIFFERENT POLICIES, PROGRAMMES AND STRATEGIES (GLOBAL ASPECT)

Policies, Programmes and strategic plans on HIV/AIDS are the foundations for any meaningful and sustained response to the epidemic. A policy provides an operating framework for people whose jobs entail prevention, treatment, care, support and generally reducing the impact of the epidemic on the population. Policies can include principles on Human Rights for all and, specifically, the rights of persons living with HIV/AIDS. They can also include strategies for reducing vulnerability to HIV/AIDS for specific groups.

A country's policy on HIV/AIDS is a useful guide to domestic and international resource allocation to support specific programs. Without a policy, those managing the response to HIV/AIDS have no sense of national direction. The policy directs the creation of strategic plans and the allocation of funds to activities aimed at achieving the stated objectives of the management of the HIV/AIDS situation

United States of America

On July 13, 2010, the White House released the National HIV/AIDS Strategy (NHAS). With a vision that United States will become a place where new HIV infections are rare and when they do occur, every person, regardless of age, gender, race/ethnicity, sexual orientation, gender identity or socio-economic circumstance, will have unfettered access to high quality, life-extending care, free from stigma and discrimination. The specific Goals of the National HIV/AIDS Strategy include reducing New HIV infections by 2015. Increasing Access to Care and Improving Health Outcomes for People Living with HIV by 2015. Reducing HIV-related health disparities and to improve access to prevention and care services for all Americans. The strategies action steps includes reducing new HIV infections, increasing access to care and improving health outcomes for people living with HIV, reducing HIV-related disparities and health inequities and achieving a more coordinated national response to the HIV epidemic

European Union

The geographical scope of the action Plan on HIV/AIDS in the EU and neighbouring countries: 2014-2016 includes EU Member States, EEA/EFTA countries and neighbouring countries, namely the EU Enlargement countries, the European Neighbourhood Policy (ENP) countries, in particular the Eastern ones bordering the EU, as well as the Russian Federation. The overall objectives of the Commission is to contribute to reducing new HIV infections across all European countries, to improve access to prevention, treatment, care and support and improving the quality of life of people living with, affected by or most vulnerable to HIV/AIDS in the European Union and neighbouring countries.

Operational action plans are structured in six key issue areas: Politics, policies and involvement of civil society, wider society and stakeholders, Targeted and combination prevention and treatment, Priority regions and settings, Priority groups, improving knowledge by promoting research for the development of new or better prevention, diagnostic and treatment solutions for HIV, co-infections and co-morbidity and regular monitoring and evaluation.

South Africa

The South African National Strategic Plan on HIV, STIs and TB 2012-2016 is a framework to guide the activities of all partners whose work is relevant to HIV, sexually transmitted infections (STIs) and TB in South Africa. It provides goals and strategies for the country's response to the three diseases during the period 2012 to 2016. The NSP will guide the development of provincial strategic implementation plans, as well as sector implementation plans. The NSP vision is based on a 20-year vision for reversing the burden of disease from HIV, STIs and TB in South Africa. It includes zero new HIV and TB infections; zero new infections due to HIV transmission from mother to child; zero preventable deaths from HIV and TB; and zero discrimination associated with HIV, STIs and TB.

The NSP has five specific goals: reducing the number of new HIV infections by half; to ensure that at least 80% of people who are eligible for treatment for HIV are receiving it. (At least 70% should be alive and still on treatment after five years); halve the number of new TB infections and deaths from TB; to ensure that the rights of people living with HIV are protected; and halve stigma related to HIV and TB.

The NSP has identified a number of strategic objectives that will help South Africa to reach these goals. These are: to address social and structural factors that drive these epidemics that influence their impact, and that affect the way we care for affected people, to prevent new HIV, STIs and TB infections through a combination of interventions, to sustain health and wellness, primarily by reducing deaths and disability from HIV, AIDS and TB and to protect human rights of people living with HIV and improve their access to justice.

The guiding principles that will underpin the revised structures will include: Access to relevant information; 'Bottom-up' governance; Accountability and responsibility; Reporting; Transparency; and Meaningful involvement of people living with HIV and TB.

The NSP has identified four core strategic enablers for effective implementation: Effective and transparent governance and institutional arrangements; Effective communication; Monitoring, evaluation and research.

Uganda

The goal of the National HIV prevention strategy for Uganda 2011-13 is to reduce new HIV infections countrywide by 30% based on the 2009 levels, which will achieve a 40% reduction of the projected new HIV infections in 2015. The strategy has specific goals that new HIV infections be reduced by 30% of the 2009 levels to achieve a 40% reduction of the projected new infections in 2015, PMTCT Rate Reduced to less than 10% by 2015 and 180,000 new HIV infections averted over 5 years. The expected outcomes are to increase coverage and utilization of HIV prevention services, increased adoption of safer sexual behaviour and reduced risky behaviours; a strengthened and sustainable enabling environment that mitigates underlying factors that drive the HIV epidemic; achieving a more coordinated HIV prevention response at all levels; strengthening information systems for HIV prevention.

The strategies and priority action includes: Increased coverage and utilization of HIV prevention services; Increased adoption of safer sexual behaviour and reduced risky behaviours; a strengthened and sustainable enabling environment that mitigates underlying factors that drive the HIV epidemic; achieving a more coordinated HIV prevention response at all levels and strengthened information systems for HIV prevention.

Monitoring and periodic evaluation of HIV prevention initiatives in this strategy will be essential to maintain an informed and strategically guided response. Progress in meeting the goals of the strategy will be reported on annually by the Uganda ADS Commission. Enhanced Monitoring and Evaluation will be necessary to ensure that HIV prevention efforts are aligned to the drivers of the epidemic based on effective approaches, and are on course to meet the targets set in the strategy.

Jamaica

The vision statement of the national HIV/AIDS policy Jamaica may 2005 is to protect the rights of all Jamaicans including those infected with and affected by HIV/AIDS and to create an enabling environment free of stigma and discrimination and providing access to prevention knowledge and skills; treatment care and support and other services.

The specific objective includes: To reduce the number of new HIV infections through the establishment of a supportive policy/ legislative environment that: To strengthen mechanisms for the treatment, care and support of persons living with and affected by HIV/AIDS through a policy and legal framework and enabling environment that: To mitigate the socio-economic impact of HIV/ AIDS on individuals, families, communities and the nation through a policy and legal framework that: To foster enabling policy regulatory and legislative environment around HIV/ AIDS issues including strengthening and sustaining a comprehensive, multi sectoral response: To affirm the rights of persons living with and affected by HIV/AIDS and the rights of those most vulnerable to HIV/AIDS through an environment that

The Guiding Principle includes: Political Leadership and Commitment; Good Governance, Transparency and Accountability; Multisectoral Approach and Partnerships; Participation; Equity; Promotion and Protection of Human Rights.

The national AIDS policy Implementation plan includes: Management and Coordination; National HIV Research Agenda; Rights and Responsibilities of Stakeholders; Monitoring, Evaluation & Review of the Policy and moreover the national HIV/AIDS Policy shall be reviewed every five years and the goal and strategies will be reviewed to ensure relevance to the national HIV/AIDS situation.

The HIV/AIDS policy and implementation plan of action includes: That all organisations/workplaces have at least designated a focal point on HIV/AIDS with a working committee representing management and employees and a PLWHA. That all organisations/ workplaces have a policy framework - guidelines or a full policy such as the National HIV/AIDS Policy, the National HIV/AIDS Workplace Policy, a Sector Policy on HIV/AIDS or an adaptation. All organisation and workplace monitor and evaluate the HIV/AIDS policies and programme implementation. Proper follow up of non-discrimination, prevention, training and Care and support services.

Thailand

The vision of Thailand National AIDS Strategy 2012-2016 is: To get to Zero New HIV Infections; to get to Zero AIDS-related Deaths; to get to Zero Stigma and Discrimination. The strategic goal includes: that new HIV infections be reduced by two-thirds; rate of vertical transmission of HIV less than 2%; Equal access to quality treatment, care, support and social protection for all people affected by HIV; AIDS related deaths reduced by half ; TB deaths among people living with HIV reduced by half; All laws and policies which obstruct equal access to prevention, treatment and care services are revised; Human Rights and gender specific needs are addressed in all HIV responses; Stigma and discrimination of PLHIV and key affected populations reduced by half

The national Strategic Direction includes: Innovation and Change; by expanding rights based and gender sensitive comprehensive prevention services for populations with risk behaviour with highest number of HIV infections; the protection of social and legal environment; Creating a sense of ownership at the local level in the expansion of prevention and control of AIDS; implement a new generation of strategic information to inform and guide the national response at all levels and to harmonize and optimize interventions and programs focusing on.

Optimization and consolidation strategy will includes: Prevention of Mother to Child Transmission (PMTCT); Prevention among Young People; Condom Programming; Blood Safety and Universal Precaution; Treatment, Care and Support ; Care and Support for Children Affected by AIDS; Stigma and Discrimination; Public Communication

Camboda

The guiding principles of the national strategic plan for comprehensive & multi-sectoral response to HIV/AIDS III (2011-2015) includes: Universal Access; Evidence based and cost-effective; Greater Involvement of People Living with or affected by HIV and AIDS (GIPA); Rights-based; Gender -equitable; Multisectoral; Linked to poverty and overall development planning.

The national strategic goals includes: To reduce the number of new HIV infections through scaled targeted prevention; To increase care and support to people living with and affected by HIV and AIDS and to alleviate the socioeconomic and human impact of AIDS on the individual, family, community and society.

The Specific Objectives and Interventions, by Strategies are: To increase coverage, quality and effectiveness of prevention interventions; to increase coverage and quality of comprehensive and integrated treatment, care and support services addressing the needs of a concentrated epidemic; to increase coverage, quality and effectiveness of interventions to mitigate the impact of HIV and AIDS; to ensure effective leadership and management by government and other actors for implementation of the national response to HIV and AIDS, at national and sub-national levels; ensure a supportive legal and public policy environment for the national response to HIV and AIDS; to ensure availability and use of strategic information for decision-making through monitoring, evaluation and research and to ensure sustained, predictable financing and cost-effective resource allocation for the national response.

China

The guiding principles of China's National Medium-and Long-Term Strategic Plan for HIV/AIDS Prevention and Control is to slow down the HIV/AIDS epidemic through substantiated prevention and control efforts and help to achieve the goal of national socio-economic development; to implement the strategies and measures, Strengthen leadership, enhance coordination among sectors and mobilize all the entire society. Implementation of a comprehensive approach, scientific research and international cooperation is actively encouraged; to strengthen health education, behavioural change and Standardize STD management; and all the prevention and control work must take the local situation and realities into consideration.

In March, 2006, the State Council of the People's Republic of China officially announced the first legislation directly aimed at controlling HIV/AIDS: the AIDS Prevention and Control Regulations. These regulations, together with the Five-Year Action Plan to Control HIV/AIDS (2006-2010), are an important step in the development of government policy related to the care and prevention of HIV/AIDS.

The Chinese government "Four Free and One Care" policy for AIDS control includes: Free antiretroviral drugs to AIDS patients who are rural residents or people without insurance living in urban areas; Free voluntary counselling and testing; Free drugs to HIV-infected pregnant women to prevent mother-to-child transmission, and HIV testing of newborn babies; Free schooling for AIDS orphans and Care and economic assistance to the households of people living with HIV/AIDS.

Hongkong

The vision of HIV/AID Strategies for Hong Kong 2012-2016 is Zero new HIV infections, zero discrimination, and zero AIDS-related deaths.

The guiding principles are: Diversified approaches are to be combined strategically based on latest evidence with regard to epidemiology, research findings and programme response to actively address the heterogeneous and evolving needs of communities at higher risk of HIV infection; Available resources are to be targeted to reduce those risk behaviours and underlying vulnerabilities of priority communities which can bring down new HIV infections; Priority areas for action are widely shared, owned and regularly reviewed by stakeholders; Services that reach marginalized communities are sensitive to their human rights; Effective responses are made sustainable, brought to scale, and are flexible enough to make continuous improvement as the situation evolves; Policies and programmes are coordinated among agencies, optimized to engage and empower community members, and guided by strategic information; The environment is conducive to universal access of HIV prevention, treatment, care and support, especially by the communities most vulnerable to HIV infection and Monitoring and evaluation forms an integral part of the local AIDS programme.

The specific goal is to sustain the reduction of new HIV/AIDS patients and ensure universal access to quality and non-discriminatory prevention, treatment, care and support services. The objectives are: to empower communities most affected by HIV to reduce their risk behaviours and underlying vulnerabilities; to ensure sustainable resources and adequate numbers of trained personnel for provision of quality and non-discriminatory services and to move towards an increasingly results-based implementation of prevention, treatment, care and support services. The strategies spell out priority areas for action which includes: scaling up HIV prevention in priority communities; maintaining holistic and quality HIV treatment, care and support; Foster an environment which supports safer sex, harm reduction and anti- discrimination; Drive strategically informed and accountable interventions and enhance partnership and capacity for an effective response within Hong Kong and the nearby region.

Australia

The vision of Australia HIV strategy 2012-15 is to work towards the virtual Elimination of HIV Transmission in NSW By 2020.

The goals and Targets by 2015 includes: to reduce the transmission of HIV among gay and other homosexually active men by 60%, and by 80% by 2020; Reduce heterosexual transmission of HIV and transmission of HIV among Aboriginal populations by 50%; Sustain the virtual elimination of mother-to-child HIV transmission; Sustain the virtual elimination of HIV transmission in the sex industry; Sustain the virtual elimination of HIV transmission among people who inject drugs; Reduce the average time between HIV infection and diagnosis from 4 ½ years to 1 ½ years; Increase to 90% the proportion of people living with HIV on antiretroviral treatment and Sustain the virtual elimination of HIV related deaths.

The strategies set out priority areas for action: Maintain high levels of safe behaviours; Intensify HIV prevention with priority populations; Improve access to the needle and syringe program; Promote HIV testing; make it easier to have an HIV test; Promote treatment uptake, make access to treatment easy; Provide treatment, care and support services in the community; Improve the health and well-being of people living with HIV; Continue to invest in surveillance and research to inform the response. The strategy also identified priority populations such as people living with HIV; Gay and other homosexually active men; Aboriginal people; Sex workers; People who inject drugs; People from culturally and linguistically diverse backgrounds. The strategy is guided by the following principles Partnership, Bipartisanship, Greater involvement of PLHA and Harm Minimization.

INDIAN CONTEXT

The National AIDS Control Program in India was prepared by the Ministry of Health and family welfare, Government of India under the aegis of National AIDS Control Organisation (NACO). During the span of time it has undergone several changes since its inception in the year 1992. The 1st NACP was initially designed for five year 1992-1997 but due to various difficulties in program, planning and implementation it was extended for another two years till 1999 when the 2nd NACP finally rolls out. The main focus of the 1st NACP was mass campaign on awareness. Likewise the 2nd NACP was also designed for five years 1999-2004 and it has undergone dramatic changes focusing on prevention intervention among targeted populations, institutional strengthening and inter sectoral collaboration. The 2nd NACP was also extended initially for two years till 2006 and was further again extended for one more year till 2007. Finally the 3rd NACP rolls out for another five years 2007-20012 with the main focus of halting and reversing the HIV/ AIDS epidemic in India by the year 2012 following the strategy of unified three ones, one Agreed Action Framework, one National HIV/AIDS Coordinating Authority and one agreed National M&E System. The National AIDS Control Program Phase- IV (2002-2017) aims to accelerate the process of reversal and further strengthen the epidemic response in India through a cautious and well defined integration process over the next five years. It continues to give emphasis on Unified three ones with additionally focusing on Quality, Innovation and Integration, partnership with comprehensive care, support and treatment. NACP IV being a very ambitious project, it didn't really take off until writing of this thesis though.

National AIDS Control Program - Phase I {(1992 - 1997)-1999}

In order to combat HIV/AIDS epidemic effectively, the Government of India established National AIDS Control Organization (NACO) in 1992. Although the 1st phase of the National AIDS Control Program was for five years, due to slow implementation in the initial period it was extended to March, 1999. The National AIDS control program phase 1 was funded by World Bank and a strong WHO Global Program on AIDS (GPA) support. The ultimate objective of the project was to slow the spread of HIV to reduce future morbidity, mortality, and the impact of AIDS by initiating and establishing a comprehensive multisectoral program.

The various components of the first phase were:

(a) Program management

(b) Intersectoral collaboration

(c) HIV and AIDS surveillance

(d) Targeted interventions among high risk groups

(e) Condom Programming

(f) Sexually Transmitted Disease (STD) Program

(g) Blood safety program

(h) Information, education and communication (I.E.C)

(i) Impact reduction

Awareness levels that were almost insignificant have increased to about 70-80% in urban areas even though the level of awareness in rural areas remains low at about 30%; Modernization and strengthening of blood banks; introduction of licensing system of blood banks and gradual phasing out of professional blood donors; and availability of good quality condoms through social marketing has made a significant increase in its use.

Despite the overwhelming rise in the awareness level of the people about HIV and AIDS it resulted in creating a fear psychosis about the virus. The experience of the past five years (1992-1997) revealed that IEC has miserably failed to meet the objectives spelt out. It can be alleged that no substantial effort has been made to reach to the general population to raise awareness, knowledge and understanding of HIV and AIDS issues even when many of the medical and paramedical staff are ignorant about the basic facts of HIV and AIDS. The impact of HIV and AIDS due to lack of proper planning and implementation of the program and lack of professionalism in it heightened the level of stigma already attached to it.

The National AIDS Control Program - Phase - II [{(1999-2004)-2006}-07]

The National AIDS control program phase 2 was sanctioned initially for 5 years (1999-2004) but was extended for two years (1999-2006) and was again extended till 2007 when the third phase finally took off. In November 1999, the second National AIDS Control Project (NACP) was launched with World Bank credit support of USD 191 million. Based on the experience gained in Tamil Nadu and a few other states along with the evolving trends of the HIV/AIDS epidemic, the focus shifted from raising awareness to changing behaviour, decentralization of program implementation at the state level and greater involvement of NGOs. The policy and strategic shift was reflected in the two key objectives of NACP II. Reducing the spread of HIV infection in India, Increasing India's capacity to respond to HIV/AIDS on a long-term basis, Achieving condom use of not less than 90%among high risk categories like commercial sex workers, truck drivers etc., and Achieving awareness level of not less than 90% among the youth and others in the reproductive age groups, Reducing blood borne diseases and transmission of HIV to less than 1% of total transmission. It supports decentralization of service delivery to the States and Municipalities and a new facilitating role for National AIDS Control Organization. Program delivery was more flexible, evidence-based and participatory to rely on local Program implementation plans. Protection of human rights by encouraging voluntary counselling and testing and discouraging mandatory testing would be a priority; it also supports structural and evidence-based annual reviews and ongoing operational research; and also encourage management reforms, such as better managed State level AIDS Control Societies and improved drug and equipment procurement practices.

Various components of NACP phase - ii includes: Prioritizing targeted interventions for populations at high risk group; Preventive interventions for the general population; Low Cost care and support for people living with HIV/AIDS; Institutional strengthening and Inter-sectoral collaboration.

While the success of NACP II could not be undermine but there are complexities to be understood. There are Complexities of the epidemic and its exact dimensions which have to be understood especially in the Northern and North Eastern states of the country. There is a frequent change of Project Directors (PDs) of State AIDS Control Societies (SACS) and other senior program managers at the state level which weakened the thrust and focus of interventions. In some highly vulnerable States, Project Directors were either saddled with additional non-HIV responsibilities or given SACS charge as additional responsibility. A large number of functional positions in the SACS remained vacant. These factors contributed to an uneven implementation of the program.

Notwithstanding a significant step-up of the overall resource availability for HIV/AIDS program, India's per capita financial investment on HIV prevention, control, care and support remains one of the lowest in the world. To scale up activities and interventions in prevention, care and treatment, a much higher level of investment is required.

The experience of NACP-I and NACP-II, consultations, studies and assessments led to a consensus on the goal, objectives and strategies for NACP-III adhering to the larger Millennium development goal.

The National AIDS Control Program Phase - III (2007-2012)

The overall goal of NACP-III is to halt and reverse the epidemic in India over the next 5 years by integrating programs for prevention, care, support and treatment. This will be achieved through a four-pronged strategy: Prevention of new infections in high risk groups and general population through: Saturation of coverage of high risk groups with targeted interventions (TIs), Scaled up interventions in the general population , Providing greater care, support and treatment to larger number of PLHA, Strengthening the infrastructure, systems and human resources in prevention, care, support and treatment program at the district, state and national level and Strengthening the nationwide Strategic Information Management System.

The specific objective is to reduce new infection as estimated in the first year of the program by: Sixty per cent (60%) in high prevalence states so as to obtain the reversal of the epidemic; and Forty per cent (40%) in the vulnerable states so as to stabilize the epidemic.

The goal, objectives and strategies of NACP-III will be informed by the following guiding principles: The unifying credo of Three Ones, i.e., one Agreed Action Framework, one National HIV/AIDS Coordinating Authority and one agreed National M&E System.

NACP-III would evolve mechanisms to be put in place at all levels to address issues related to human rights and ethics. Particular focus would be on the fundamental rights of PLHA and their active involvement as important partners in prevention, care, support and treatment initiatives. Civil society representation and participation in planning and implementation of NACP-III would receive priority since it is essential for promoting social ownership and community involvement. Creation of an enabling environment wherein those infected and affected by HIV could lead a life of dignity. This will be the corner-stone of all interventions. Stigma and discrimination associated with HIV/AIDS, which continues to pose a big challenge to policy planners and program implementers in prevention, care and treatment efforts will be aggressively addressed. Having regard to the spirit behind "universal access", NACP-III will scale up efforts and activities for providing HIV prevention, care, support, and treatment services. For making the implementation mechanism more responsive, proactive and dynamic, the HRD strategy of NACO and SACS will be based on qualification, competence, commitment and continuity. Strategic and program interventions will be evidence-based and result-oriented with scope for innovations and flexibility. Priority will be accorded to specific local contexts.

NACP-III seeks to learn from the lessons of the previous two phases of program implementation and build on the strengths thereof. Its priorities and thrust areas have been drawn up accordingly and include the following:

Considering that more than 99% of the population in the country is free from infection, NACP-III will place the highest priority on preventive efforts to all types of population while, at the same time, seeking to integrate prevention with care, support and treatment. Prevention needs of children will be addressed through universal provision of PPTCT services. Children who are infected will be assured access to paediatric ART. It will also make efforts to address the needs of persons infected and affected by HIV, especially children. It will invest in community care centres to provide psycho-social support, outreach services, referrals and palliative care. It will work with other agencies involved in vulnerability reduction such as women's groups, youth groups, trade unions etc. to integrate HIV prevention into their activities. Mainstreaming and partnerships will be the key approach to facilitate multi-sectoral response engaging a wide range of stakeholders. Private sector, civil society organizations, PLHA networks and government departments would all play crucial role in prevention, care, support, treatment and service delivery. Technical and financial resources of the development partners will be leveraged to achieve the objectives of the program.

d) The National AIDS Control Program Phase- IV (2012-2017)

The aim of NACP IV is to accelerate the process of reversal and further strengthen the epidemic response in India through a cautious and well defined integration process over the next five years.

The goal is to accelerate reversal and integrate response. The objectives are: to reduce new infections by 50% (2007 Baseline of

NACP III); to provide comprehensive care and support to all persons living with HIV/AIDS and treatment services for all those who require it.

The key strategies includes: Intensifying and consolidating prevention services, with a focus on HRGs and vulnerable population; Increasing access and promoting comprehensive care, support and treatment; Expanding IEC services for (a) general population and (b) high risk groups with a focus on behaviour change and demand generation; Building capacities at national, state, district and facility levels and Strengthening Strategic Information Management Systems.

The Guiding principles for NACP - IV will continue to be: Continued emphasis on three ones - one Agreed Action Framework, one National HIV/AIDS Coordinating Authority and one Agreed National M&E System; Equity; Gender; Respect for the rights of the PLHIV; Civil society representation and participation; Improved public private partnerships; Evidence based and result oriented programme implementation.

The Cross-cutting Areas of Focus will be on Quality, Innovation, Integration, Leveraging Partnerships, Stigma and Discrimination. Key priorities under NACP- IV are:

- Preventing new infections by sustaining the reach of current interventions and effectively addressing emerging epidemics;
- Prevention of Parent to Child transmission; Focusing on IEC strategies for behaviour change in HRG, awareness among general population and demand generation for HIV services;
- Providing comprehensive care, support and treatment to eligible PLHIV;
- Reducing stigma and discrimination through Greater involvement of PLHA (GIPA);
- De-centralizing rollout of services including technical support;
- Ensuring effective use of strategic information at all levels of programme;

- Building capacities of NGO and civil society partners especially in states with emerging epidemics;
- Integrating HIV services with health systems in a phased manner;
- Mainstreaming of HIV/ AIDS activities with all key central/ state level Ministries/ departments will be given a high priority and resources of the respective departments will be leveraged.
- Social protection and insurance mechanisms for PLHIV will be strengthened.

Some New Initiatives under NACP-IV includes: Differential strategies for districts based on data triangulation with due weightage to vulnerabilities; Scale up of programmes to target key vulnerabilities a. Scale up of Opioid Substitution Therapy (OST) for IDUs b. Scale up and strengthening of Migrant Interventions at Source, Transit & Destinations including roll out of Migrant Tracking System for effective outreach c. Establishment and scale up of interventions for Transgenders (TGs) by bringing in community participation and focused strategies to address their vulnerabilities d. Employer-Led Model for addressing vulnerabilities among migrant labour e. Female Condom Programme; Scale up of Multi-Drug Regimen for Prevention of Parent to Child Transmission (PPTCT) in keeping with international protocols; Social protection for marginalised populations through mainstreaming and earmarking budgets for HIV among concerned government departments; Establishment of Metro Blood Banks and Plasma Fractionation Centre; Launch of Third Line ART and scale up of first and second Line ART and Demand promotion strategies specially using mid-media, e.g., National Folk Media Campaign & Red Ribbon Express and buses [in convergence with the National Rural Health Mission(NRHM

NORTH EAST LEVEL

The North Eastern Region, comprising the seven States of Assam, Arunachal Pradesh, Manipur, Meghalaya, Mizoram, Nagaland and Tripura, is an extensive area, (about 7.8% of India's land area) with 3.7% of total population. It is strategically located, bound by Chinese occupied Tibet and Bhutan to the North and West, Myanmar to the East and Bangladesh to the West and South, connected to mainland India by a narrow corridor in North Bengal. Specifically, the States of Mizoram, Manipur, Nagaland and Arunachal Pradesh share long borders with Myanmar to the East, across hilly, forested, thinly populated terrain. This critical location has had major implications for HIVAIDS problem in the North Eastern Region.

HIV surveillance was initiated first at Guwahati Medical College and thereafter at Regional Medical College, Imphal, and other places in 1986. Beginning with the first case of HIV detected in Manipur, there has been a steep rise in number of cases detected and prevalence of HIV among specific risk groups in certain States of the Region. The startling escalation in number of HIV cases led to the discovery of IV drug abuse as the chief cause of the HIV problem in the Region.

One high HIV prevalence states Nagaland and low prevalence state of Assam has been included in the selection for policy discussion.

The Assam State HIV/AIDS Prevention and Control Policy aims to halt and reverse the AIDS epidemic in the State to zero transmission rate and to reduce the impact of the epidemic at all levels of general population. The specific objectives of the policy are:

- To reiterate strongly the Government's firm commitment to prevent the spread of HIV infection and to reduce personal and social impact;
- To ensure right to privacy and confidentiality of people living with HIV/AIDS (PLHA);
- To ensure an environment free of discrimination for people living with HIV/AIDS and protection of human rights, including right to access healthcare system both at the government and private sectors;
- To ensure prevention of hospital acquired infections for a safe environment; To ensure information, treatment and support to the people under care and custody of the State;

- To strengthen safe blood transfusion system both at the Government and private institutions;To mainstream AIDS Prevention and Control Programme with partnership development;
- To ensure HIV/AIDS related information, education and communication (IEC) at all levels;
- To promote strategies for risk reduction from drug addiction and unsafe sex;
- To prevent women, children and other socially weaker groups from becoming vulnerable to HIV infection by improving health education, legal status and economic empowerment;
- To promote mapping and surveillance for adequate intervention and estimation of the burden of infection in the State;
- To promote proper Monitoring and Evaluation system and to ensure accountability;
- To develop appropriate legal framework.

The State of Assam has been included as it is highly vulnerable state for HIV transmission because of the following reasons:

- It is the gate-way of North-eastern states;
- It is surrounded by two high prevalence states of Manipur and Nagaland;
- Large number of female migrants from other north-eastern states, West Bengal, Nepal who has come to Assam for Employment and has taken to sex work;
- High-prevalence of other Sexual Transmitted Infections, stigma and social discrimination, inequity, high prevalence of risky sexual behavior among young people, existence of mobile and hidden nature of female sex workers, drug abuse, injecting drug use, illegal drug trafficking, etc are also responsible for increased vulnerability of the State.

Nagaland as per 2014 Sentinel Surveillance Report has recorded the highest prevalence of HIV & AIDS in the country with an alarming ratio of 0.88 per cent against country's figure stands at 0.37 per cent. The state has 10 'A' category districts. It has now been 17 years since the first HIV/AIDS positive case was detected in the year 1990 amongst the IDUs by ICMR. The programme is implemented through Nagaland State AIDS Control Society headed by Project Director and 3 Deputy Directors and other supporting officers and staff totaling 60, with the launching of NACP III, There are 14 NGO doing Targeted Intervention Programme in the State.

The goal is to halt and reverse the HIV/AIDS epidemic. The objectives include:

- Prevention of new infection in the high risk groups and general population through;
- Saturation of coverage of high risk groups with targeted intervention (TIs);
- Scaled up intervention in general population;
- Providing greater care and support and treatment to the large number of people living with HIV/AIDS;
- Strengthening the infrastructure, system and human resource in prevention, care, support, & treatment programmes at the district, state and National level;
- Strengthening a nation - wide Strategic Information Management System.

Over the years the trend of epidemic has moved from high risk behavioral group to general population and from urban to rural areas. Sexual routine of transmission has taken predominance with 78.73% followed by infected needles and syringes with 12.21 %.

Surveillance report shows that the most vulnerable population is in the age group between 15-29 years.

State AIDS Council: State AIDS Council has been formed with Chief Minister as the Chairman. Nagaland Legislative Forum Secretariat has been established with a consultant. 58 Legislatures have contributed Rs. 50,000/- (Rupees Fifty Thousand) each from Local Area Development Plan fund (LAPDF) for Nagaland Legislative Forum activities.

Eleven DACPUs have been formed which will operate within the District Health Society sharing the administrative health financial structure of NRHM and will implement the programme at district level.

Manipur

As the first few cases of HIV infection of the country were reported in 1986, the Manipur State Government also took serious note of the problem and initiated a series of important measures to tackle the epidemic. The first HIV/AIDS cases in Manipur were detected in1989 from a blood samples collected from among IDU's in 1988. With the formation of the high-powered National AIDS Committee in 1986, Government of India launched National AIDS Control Program in 1987. In the year 1989 with the support of WHO, many other activities were initiated which were mainly focused on the reinforcement of program management capacities as well as targeted IEC and Surveillance activities. Actual preventive activities like implementation of IDU focused prevention intervention, education and awareness program, blood safety measures, control of hospital infection, condom promotion to prevent HIV/AIDS, strengthening of clinical services for both STD and HIV/AIDS gained momentum only in 1992.

Commitment of the state for development with other key societal actors being willing participant (i.e. political settlement is committed to development) for HIV/AIDS mitigation. Capacity of the state to implement policies effectively and this capacity being determined by other constituent capacities like the Institutional, technical and political. State AIDS Cells were created in Manipur for effective implementation and management of National AIDS Control Program. In 1996 the Manipur State AIDS Cell (MSACS) became Manipur State AIDS Control Society registered under Societies Act and it became an autonomous body with objectives of reducing the spread of HIV infection in the state and to increase the state capacity to deal with the epidemic in the long term. Most of the programmes launched in the field of HIV/AIDS are with the help of MSAC, NACO and NGOs. The external agencies gave more emphasis on Prevention with minimum attention on treatment, care and support.

For combating the menace of HIV/AIDS in Manipur, Manipur State AIDS Policy 1996 was launched with following objectives: a) to prevent the spread of HIV infection, both at the community at large and in the health care environment. b) To promote better understanding of HIV infection in order to protect and support those who are at risk of or vulnerable to infection. c) To ensure that treatment and support services both for those infected with HIV and for their family are easily available and accessible. d) To ensure that services are efficient, effective and evaluated. e) To mobilize and unify intersectoral action, community initiatives and NGO/CBO support network for better co-operation among the participating agencies against AIDS.

The State AIDS Policy has policies on various dimensions such as:

a) Policies on Information Education and Communication,

b) Policy on school AIDS education,

c) Policy on Blood Safety,

d) Policy on Medical Care,

e) Policy on Std and Reproductive Health,

f) Policy on Drug Abuse Treatment Service,

g) Policy on Hospital Infection Control,

h) Policy on Intervention Measures,

i) Policy on Employment,

j) Policy on Antibody Testing,

k) Policy on Confidentiality,

l) Policy in the Prisons/Jails,

m) Policy on Social Service Research,

n) Policy on Non-Discrimination Provision,

o) Policy on Training and

p) Policy on Appropriate Legal Framework.

In order to facilitate speedy and proper implementation of the AIDS control programme, the State Government created appropriate bodies such as State AIDS Committee (SAC) with State Empowered Committee (SEC), and State Level AIDS Co-ordination Committee (SCC). It also created grass root infrastructure by creating District AIDS Committee (DAC). Despite all these efforts, the situation is getting worse.

STATEMENT OF THE PROBLEMS

The growing menace created by the HIV and AIDS (human immunodeficiency virus/acquired immunodeficiency syndrome) has alarmed not only the public health officials but also the general community. HIV and AIDS are more than a health problem and its impact reaches far beyond the health sector with severe economic and social consequences. HIV and AIDS affect individuals, families and communities at the micro-level whereas it equally affects the various sectors of the economy at the macro-level.

Attention must be paid to HIV/AIDS related activities as part of overall development policy. It is essential to have impact on the factors that sustain the HIV epidemic and contribute to its progress and to integrate the social and health policy goals and resource requirement that the epidemic calls for more clearly into development policy. Factors that give rise to the epidemic accelerate its spread and makes its effect worse like lack of institutional capacity, poverty, low level of education, social inequality, conflicts, discrimination, gender inequality and both sex trade and sexual violence. HIV/AIDS has its widespread effects on society, culture, individuals and families.

Worldwide, most of those infected by HIV/AIDS are working men and women, the mainstay of families, communities, enterprises and economies. The epidemic is changing the dynamics of the labour force — experienced, skilled workers are dying, children are being forced to work and a greater burden is being placed on women.

The traditional domestic and nurturing roles of women mean that they bear most of the burden of care. This not only adds to their workload but also undermines the vital productive, reproductive and community roles they play. According to UNDCP, 2002 Poverty contributes to the spread of HIV, and women make up 70% of the world's poor, reflecting their limited access to employment, property, credit and income.

LIMITATIONS OF THE STUDY

Most of the organization which was studied has a poor documentation reports, this compels the researcher to dig out information through primary sources. Due to constant general strikes most of the organisation couldn't functions their day to day activities according to their monthly plans. There was difficulty accessing the IDU's in such situation where police vigilance was high. Police was acting as moral guardians to the society. There was difficulty in accessing Assembly proceedings report as the said document was available only up to the year 2010 though Assembly sitting was continuously held up to date. Content analysis of the said report has been done only up to 2010 as government records were not available.

LITERATURE REVIEW AND RESEARCH METHODOLOGY

To have an in-depth knowledge of policies, programmes and Interventions of the AIDS pandemic, it is important to take stock of the information available. HIV and AIDS is an extensively researched area. The last few decades has brought forth research from professionals representing Medicine, Psychology, Sociology, Economics, Political Science, Anthropology and others. Doubtless to say these have added to building a strong knowledge base. It would be of interest to look at the literature available under three heads: a) Policies b) Programmes c) Interventions

Policies

Wouters E. et al 2010, reviewed the HIV/AIDS policies in South Africa. The response and management of HIV/AIDS pandemic in

South Africa is, to a large extent case of lost opportunities. According to them the country has encountered one of the worst epidemics in the world; consecutive national AIDS strategies have been repeatedly marked by failure over almost three decades. Understandably, South Africa's most recent HIV/AIDS policy, the HIV & AIDS and STI Strategic Plan for South Africa, 2007-2011 (National Strategic Plan-NSP), has been greeted with general acclaim. However, what are its real prospects of success against the backdrop of the repeated failures of the past? The objective of the review was to systematically identify the core reasons for past policy failures. Using a comprehensive analytical framework, this article presents a systematic review of the literature on post apartheid AIDS policy in South Africa. The analysis demonstrates that a complex interplay among the content, context, actors and process of AIDS policy created a gap between policy making and policy implementation. Secondly they evaluated that the chances of success of the current NSP by examining both the policy-making phase and the resulting policy document in light of the reasons for past policy failures. The analysis shows that the NSP contains dynamic and comprehensive policy content, sensitive to the socio-economic and cultural dimensions of HIV/AIDS. Wouters adds that many of the political actors who hampered treatment implementation in the past, and who deepened the gap between government and civil society, are still in office. Also monetary and human resource shortages also create a policy context that is unsuitable for the implementation of a comprehensive HIV/AIDS strategy, as envisaged in the NSP. Finally, the health system restrictions have a clear negative impact on the process of policy implementation. Without the mobilization of people living with HIV/AIDS and their communities, the NSP will be ineffective in bridging the gap between policy intentions and policy implementation.

M. Shanmugam, K. et al., 2008 says like most other countries, India is also following an HIV prevention programs predominantly focusing on behaviour change at the individual level overlooking both the enabling environment needed for sustaining healthy behaviors as well as the broader needs and rights of vulnerable communities. For HIV prevention programs to succeed, a holistic approach towards improving the health and rights of vulnerable populations and people living with HIV and AIDS is crucial.

Genuine participation of affected communities is considered a best practice when making HIV/AIDS policy and decisions (F.C. Iskandar et al., 2008). The lesson learned in the study was that communities demonstrated that, when approached they actively respond and contribute to policy and decision making processes. More than 66% of respondents represent different networks of PLHIV, NGOs and CBOs. The effective online consultation was open, inclusive and efficient. Consultation for community engagement is possible, by ensuring that affected communities have practical platforms to inform national and regional HIV processes; it adds value to the existing body of evidence and increases mutual accountability and ownership between stakeholders.

According to Aruldas V et al 2008, a policy to guide a Churches response to HIV/AIDS is complex, because it is not only an expression that guides proposed actions, but also represents a value statement that guides the lives and actions of its individual members. The review bring forth that ideology, culture, social and other contextual differences do influence policies/declarations, even when they are developed by groups (in this case churches) belonging to the same religion. A reference framework based on experiences of similar organisations helps enrich the policy formulation process.

Programs of NGOs, GOs, FBOs

There are various programs followed by nongovernmental, governmental organisation, faith based organisations and other community based organisations. Kapur S., 1996, discussed the programmes developed by The Voluntary Health Association of India (VHAI), with financial support and technical advice from the European Commission. The program began in January 1995. Its overall goal was to strengthen the capacities of nongovernmental organizations (NGOs) in initiating and developing HIV/AIDS interventions at the grass-roots level. Program strategies include capacity building within NGOs for effective HIV/AIDS efforts, primary prevention of HIV/sexually transmitted disease (STD) transmission through information and education and promotion of safer sex, promotion of condom use, and improvement of STD control in primary health care, and advocacy and social mobilization in support of persons affected by HIV/AIDS. VHAI first invited project proposals from NGOS in Manipur, Assam, West Bengal, Bihar, Kerala, and Andhra Pradesh. Then it held a workshop for interested NGOs on policy and funding criteria. 24 NGOs were selected in the first round from all the above states, except Andhra Pradesh. The intended audiences included youth, women, migrant workers, intravenous drug users, commercial sex workers, tribals, and students. The selected projects consisted of awareness generation, needle exchange, blood safety, condom promotion, and counseling. Training programs addressed project management, counseling, and training of health personnel (medical practitioners, health workers, peer educators, and paramedical workers). State-specific communication strategies involved traditional and folk media, a condom key chain, and workshops for journalists, and meetings with members of the Legislative Assembly. VHAI is developing a comprehensive communication package for lobbying and advocacy activities. The May-June 1996 mid-term evaluation found that the program helped state VHAs to work more closely with member NGOS and non-member groups and that NGOs did become familiar with HIV/STD prevention and control. NGOS had inadequate experience in project management. NGOs were able to mobilize communities, to take on innovative interventions and to network effectively.

Ucheaga DN and Hartwig KA., 2010 made a formative research on HIV/AIDS prevention messages, activities and policies within six religious institutions in Cross River State, Nigeria, at urban and rural sites. The findings indicate that religious organisations are already playing a role in HIV prevention but their responses are not uniform. Public health organisations and policy-makers should be aware of these denominational differences as they engage with religious institutions and leaders in HIV prevention and care

Some of the major programs of the faith based organization in India are

- Counseling support groups for people living with HIV/AIDS and their families

- Support groups for educating local communities about HIV/AIDS
- Peer education programs which aims at prevention of HIV and sexually transmitted infections
- Income-generation and vocational training programs for people living with HIV/AIDS and their dependents
- Care and support programs for children orphaned by AIDS
- Voluntary counseling and testing services

Examples of a faith based organization intervention programmes in Manipur with special reference to Christianity:

- Children advocacy programme:
- Youth Support Structures at Community level:
- Parents Capacity Building:
- Community Capacity Building (leaders)
- Peer Approaches

According to studies conducted by Bansal R.K., et al 1998, concludes that the long distance truck crews are at high risk of contracting and transmitting STDs and HIV on account of their high risk sexual behaviours. The study indicates the necessity of changing the behaviour of the truck crew in favour of safer sexual practices. The paper addresses this important issue of developing an intervention to decrease the risk of contraction of STDs, including HIV, by encouraging the use of condoms by the method of applying psycho-social theories, which aim at changing behaviours of the target group.

The paper discusses the development of an intervention to decrease risk of sexually transmitted diseases (STDs) and HIV/AIDS of the truck crew of India using the "Applying Theories" model in promoting condom use. The study shows that truck crews were at a high risk of infection and transmission of both STDs and HIV on account of their high-risk sexual behaviors. Moreover, the study indicated the need for behavior change in favor of safer sexual practices. This document developed a working model to solve the health educational problems of a truck crew through the application of psychosocial theories. The discussion was outlined as follows: 1) problem to problem definition; 2) provisional explanations; 3) theoretical explanations; 4) additional research; and 5) solutions. Generally, solutions generated include health education services for the truck crew, training of doctors who attend to this population group, as well as ensuring condom availability at the halting places of truckers.

Stigma against persons living with HIV/AIDS (PLHA) is a barrier to seeking prevention education, HIV testing, and care. Social capital has been reported as an important factor influencing HIV prevention and social support upon infection. Sivaram S., et al 2009, study explored the associations between social capital and stigma among men and women who are patrons of wine shops or community-based alcohol outlets in Chennai. The findings suggest that seeking partnerships with existing organizations and involving health care providers in future interventions may be explored as a strategy in community-based prevention interventions.

The findings of the study suggest that there is an urgent need to improve the coverage of services to those at-risk populations, as the worldwide coverage of HIV prevention, treatment, and care services in IDU populations is still very low.

Intervention

According to the study conducted by Mirante, E. 1993, about 25% of India's HIV positive cases come from the northeast states of Manipur, Mizoram, and Nagaland, which have only 3% of the country's total population. The reason is access to Burmese heroin just over the border, which is poorly monitored. The Meiteis, Kukis, and Nagas ethnic groups are known for their young people's involvement with drug use in urban as well as rural areas. True rehabilitation programs are in small numbers. The traffic of heroin must also be monitored so that the rate of addiction levels off and the rate of HIV infection from sharing needles levels off as well.

The study conducted by Gammelgaard. J., et al 1992, shows Infection with the human immunodeficiency virus (HIV) is spreading rapidly among injection drug users (IDUs), particularly in countries of the Golden Triangle where Myanmar (Burma), Thailand, and Laos converge and the pure heroin China White is refined. Thailand, Myanmar, Hong Kong, Malaysia, Singapore, the southern provinces of China, and the northeastern states of India viz Mizoram, Manipur and Nagaland are affected. The present study notes an increasing shift to the use of injected drugs and argues that the lack of coherent policies against using injected drugs is sure to have an effect on the HIV/AIDS transmission rates in Asia. Since the infection rates have become so high among certain IDU groups, it is probable that the infection will continue to increase in frequency as well as spread to the wives and unborn children of IDUs.

According to Sarkar, S et al., 1995, In India, there is a steep increase in the prevalence of HIV (0% to 50% within six months) among the IDUs has been reported in Manipur, a north eastern state in 1990. This article details the role of injection drug us in the increase of HIV infection in Manipur. It concludes that behavior in needle sharing is not influenced by HIV knowledge or the educational programs being implemented.

According to Panda, S., L. Bijaya, et al. (2001), In India, drug use is seen predominantly as a problem among men. This study attempts to address the interface between drug use and sex work among women drug users in Manipur and the prevalence of HIV, hepatitis B and other sexually transmitted infections in them. The article discusses the possible links between sex work, drug use and rates of HIV or hepatitis infection. It finds that HIV rates among IDUs are much higher than that of non-IDUs. However, the incidence of hepatitis infection was similar between the two groups, which suggest that hepatitis infection may be related to sexual practices rather than injection drug use since most of the women reported having sex with non-regular partners for money or drugs.

Hangzo, C, et al. (1997), conducted a study on outreach interventions using ex-IDUs to inform and educate their peers about HIV/AIDS prevention measures have been found to be effective in the United States and other developed countries. While HIV/AIDS prevention programmes targeting IDUs have also been implemented in a number of developing countries, very little information is available on the process of implementation of these programmes. This paper attempts to document some of this knowledge by describing the implementation process of an outreach intervention targeting IDUs in a small town—Churachandpur—with high injection drug use and high HIV infection rates, in the north-eastern state of Manipur. The paper describes the barriers encountered in implementing the outreach and how these barriers were minimized. In conclusion, the paper makes the case for targeting outreach to the larger community before targeting the IDUs. This paper describes the barriers encountered in implementing HIV/AIDS prevention interventions among IDUs, such as discrimination and a lack of existing services. It describes an outreach effort targeted towards IDUs in Churachandpur, and makes the case for targeting outreach to the larger community before targeting IDUs specifically.

Eicher, A.D, et al. (2000), conducted a study which aimed to measure risk behaviours and seroprevalence of HIV and hepatitis C virus in IDUs in Manipur, North-East India, and evaluate the impact of the recently established Syringe and Needle Exchange Program (SNEP). The SNEP program distributed sterile syringes and condoms, as well as collected used needles and syringes from registered clients. Only 42% of the IDUs surveyed were in contact with the SNEP. Results showed a positive association between condom use and SNEP contact.

According to Sarkar, S., et al. (1993), In India, a steep increase in the prevalence of HIV (0% to 50% within six months) among the IDUs has been reported in Manipur, a north eastern state in 1990. In spite of large scale intervention program like educational campaign and widespread voluntary HIV testing in this state, the infection has quickly spread to the heterosexual population at large. The authors determine that although there has been decline in risk behavior among IDUs, analysis reveals that unsafe needle sharing behavior is not influenced by increased knowledge of HIV transmission, educational status, history of HIV testing, or serostatus of the individual.

Bhagat, R. (2002), on online newspaper article describes the overall HIV/AIDS situation in Manipur. It discusses the connection between IDUs and the disease, as well as NGOs in Manipur acting on AIDS issues, and the consequences of needle sharing.

Riehman, K.S. (1996), paper which is prepared for policy research report for policy consideration is a basic document on the connection between HIV/AIDS and injecting drug use. It presents an overview of levels of HIV infection among drug users in various countries, and discusses the role of the IDU population in introducing HIV into the general population (IDUs as a "bridge population"), the factors influencing the global diffusion of heroin and injecting drug use, practices that facilitate the spread of HIV among IDUs, and possible interventions to reduce HIV transmission among IDUs.

Gaps if any

As of now there is no analytical review available of the national and states HIV/AIDS policies in India. Policies and programs are made for a specific period of time. Often times there are gap in the linkage of one policy to the next. In India there have been four time bound HIV/AIDS policies, NACP I, II, III and IV. However these policies, their inbuilt programmes and strategies have not been studied across all states in India which made it difficult to make comparisons between the previous programmes and the current ongoing programmes to draw a meaningful conclusion. Needless to state that scientific documents on program review and comparisons are important for several reasons. Firstly, in terms of assisting the different states to design effective and efficient interventions for curbing the epidemic in their regard; secondly, the progression of the HIV/AIDS epidemic in each state is different. This provides us with a unique opportunity for learning from those countries and states that have dealt with the epidemic for a longer period. It is important to learn and to share experiences of different state of the country in the fight against HIV/AIDS. Thus, there is clearly a need to scientifically document this crucial data in our country. Also there are no documented reports of faith based organizations their interest except for the Christian based and the Catholic in particular.

THE PRESENT STUDY

The present study aims to critically review the policy, programmes and their strategy for HIV/AIDS mitigation in a high prevalent state i.e Manipur. It also pays attention to the role of Civil Societies and F.B.O in the region. The present study on HIV/AIDS was conducted in Imphal by following a holistic view of the program, its approach and processes by focusing upon all the actors. Given the situation in Manipur, the location of the proposed study, Imphal contributed the highest number of People Living with HIV and AIDS (PLWHA) among the nine district of Manipur (Manipur State Aids Control Society). Moreover there has not been any research on the social and cultural context or the modalities of program implementation and various roles of actors and stake holders in HIV and AIDS Mitigation

RATIONALE OF THE STUDY

A comprehensive study is being carried out on the program implementation and impact of HIV and AIDS intervention in Manipur. It takes a holistic view of the programme, its approach and processes by focusing upon all the actors. Given the situation in Manipur, the location of the study, Imphal contributed the highest number of People Living with HIV and AIDS (PLWHA) among the nine district of Manipur (Manipur State Aids Control Society). Moreover there has not been any research on the social and cultural context or the modalities of program implementation and various roles of actors and stake holders in HIV and AIDS Mitigation

OBJECTIVES

It goes without saying that in HIV and AIDS mitigation not only the governmental organisation but a very large number of nongovernmental organisation have been reaching out with services to those vulnerable and those suffering alongside. Faith based organization's have shown their marked contribution. Each and every program and its service delivery are affected by a number of factors: The policy formulation, the program implementation and its operational modalities such as availability of funds, presence of skilled and trained functionaries etc. Not only is this, the political leaders and their commitment to this cause of HIV and AIDS prevention and management an aspect of great importance. The present study aims to look into all these aspects and develop an insight into the overall commitment of various actors in HIV and AIDS mitigation. The study was conducted based on the following research questions and objectives:

RESEARCH QUESTIONS

1. What is the contribution of different stakeholders in HIV/AIDS Mitigation?
2. To what extent the government is committed to HIV/AIDS mitigation?
3. Are the beneficiaries content with the services and schemes provided?
4. Did the present Policies, Programmes and Strategies serve best its purposes?

Specific objectives of the study:

1. To study and examine the existing HIV Policies, Programmes and Strategies in Manipur.
2. To analyse the modalities of program implementation by the Government and Non-Governmental Organisations.
3. To understand the political commitment of political leaders in HIV/AIDS mitigation.
4. To study beneficiaries perception of services rendered by Government and Non-Governmental Organisations.
5. To suggest the role of professional social workers in implementing prevention, care and support programmes in the field of HIV/AIDS.

OPERATIONAL DEFINITIONS

a) **HIV**: Human Immunodeficiency Virus

b) **AIDS**: Acquired Immuno Deficiency Syndrome

c) **Mitigating**: Lessening, toning down or containing the spread of HIV and AIDS

d) **Actors**: The various stake holders, government and non governmental organisations, faith based organisation in mitigation of HIV and AIDS

e) **Process**: Course of action taken to achieve certain goal

RESEARCH METHODOLOGY

Since the objectives of the study demands, the scholar used Descriptive Research Design. Descriptive research is used to obtain information concerning the current status of the phenomena to describe "what exists" with respect to variables or conditions in a situation. It also relates to those studies which are concerned with describing the characteristics of a particular individuals or groups. The present studies were concerned with specific predictions, narration of facts and concerning individuals, groups or situations and it was descriptive in nature. The study were also concerned with whether certain variables are associated with something else, it was also diagnostic in nature.

The study uses both Quantitative and Qualitative method

The researchers while using qualitative approach captured what people have to say in their own words. In contrast to it Quantitative approach focuses on objective and standardised means of inquiry and application of statistical analysis for attainment of objectivity and generalizations.

Universe and Sampling Design

The universe of the study was Imphal the capital city of Manipur. Imphal was subdivided into two districts, Imphal east and Imphal West. The researcher intends to use Non-Probability Purposive sampling and Snowball Sampling techniques. Imphal west being an administrative centre and more over 65% of the Imphal nongovernmental organization are functioning here, so the researcher selected 8 organisations from Imphal west District and 4 organisations from Imphal east District which are functional for the last five years. In order to minimize any biasness in selecting the sample, records and data's were first verified of the performance of the organisations for the last five years. There are forty nine (49) Non Governmental organisations working in the field of HIV and AIDS in Imphal area where the research Scholar carried out his research. Out of the 12 organisations 5 beneficiaries, 2 field workers, 1 administrative heads from each organisation were selected.

Knowing the importance of the roles played by Faith based organisations in the prevention of HIV/AIDS in the world, 4 leaders from the type were included in the sample. From the government 8 (Eight) MLA's from various portfolios were interviewed to find out the political commitment in the issue of health in general and HIV/AIDS in Particular. Three (3) representatives each from MSACS and ICMR Imphal unit were also interviewed. A total of 6 representatives from women organization, All Manipur Anti Drugs Association and a Notable person (Paramedical or Scholar) in the field were also interviewed. Due care was taken while selecting persons from social work background as they are the one who best experience the roles and responsibilities, any fallacy and loopholes in the policies, Programs and implementation. The sampling detail is given below in the form of a table.

List of governmental and non-governmental organization and various stake holders included in the sample

	Imphal West	Imphal East	Total
Non Governmental Organisation	8	4	12X8=96
Manipur State AIDS Control Society	3	-	3
ICMR Imphal Unit	3	-	3
Faith Based Organisation	3	1	4
Political Leaders	-	-	8
All Manipur Anti Drugs Association			2
Meira Paibis			2
Notable persons in the field of HIV and AIDS			2
Total			120

Detail Break up of Individuals interviewed in the Non Governmental Organisation

	No. of Organisa-tions	No. of Indivi-duals in each organization	Total
Beneficiaries	12	5	12X5=60
Organisational Functionaries	12	2	12X2=24
Administrative heads	12	1	12X1=12
Total			96

DATA COLLECTION

Primary data

Primary sources were employed as some of the objectives were answered through primary data. So the research Scholar uses interview schedule, interview guide, questionnaire and structured observation as method to collect information's and data's.

Secondary data

Few researchers had cautioned the limitation of secondary data as inconsistency, under, above or biased reporting so that HIV/AIDS implementing agency or the government could get some foreign grant by getting public sympathy. However the importance of secondary sources couldn't be undermined so the researcher collected data and compile a variety of secondary data source from, UNAIDS, USAID, UNDP, WHO, Population council etc. AVERT websites, CDC Websites, National AIDS control organisation websites, State AIDS policy sites, National, International news paper, Journals, Local Paper, reports from the queries and discussions on HIV/AIDS in the state assembly 1996-2007 and local self government institutions, Network of Positive people, organisation, government and non-governmental organisation and various actors (Stake Holders) in Manipur.

TOOLS OF DATA COLLECTION

For this study, the researcher used various ways and means of data collections to suit the representatives and personnel's from various fields. Since the issue is a highly sensitive matter, where talking about sex is still a taboo in the Indian society, due care was taken to protect the interest and identity of the beneficiaries and also various stake holders involved in it.

Interview Schedule

The interview schedule means the use of a set of predetermined questions and of highly standardized techniques of recording. Thus, the interviewer in a structured interview follows a rigid procedure laid down, asking questions in a form and order prescribed. Interview scheduled was prepared for the beneficiaries and the field level workers. While administering the schedule, the interviewer can probe specific answers and the questions can be repeated, rephrased on the spot in order to explain the question and get an accurate response.

Information was collected from the beneficiaries and the field workers regarding the demographic data or the socio economic background, the nature of their problem for which their accessing services, their perceived benefits and their reported difficulties in accessing these services etc.

i) Demographic Data related to the Beneficiaries and the field workers-Name, age, sex, location, educational/professional qualifications, annual income, marital status etc.

ii) Commitment to their job and the issue of mitigation of HIV and AIDS in particular

iii) Awareness related to issues of HIV and AIDS

Interview Guide

Interview guide was also prepared for Political actors at State legislature, for civil society representative like Faith Based Organisation, Administrative heads, Notable persons from nongovernmental organisation and governmental bodies. Interview guide is a step by step guideline for the interviewer so that he does not miss out any important matter.

Content analysis

The method of content analysis is being used to collect information and data especially of legislative questions and Minutes and other forms of records at local level. Since content analysis is a research techniques used to objectively and systematically make inferences about the intentions, attitudes, and values of individuals by identifying specified characteristics in textual messages. The unobtrusive nature of content analysis makes it well suited for strategic research like the one the researcher uses with parliamentary and legislature debate. The framework chosen for the purpose is simple and general, employing only a few basic concepts: The data as communicated to the researcher, the context of the data, using knowledge to partition the seen reality, the use of frequencies for deriving greater and larger meaning.

ANALYSIS OF RESULTS

The data after collection was processed and analyzed by coding, classification and tabulation of the collected data. Appropriate software, Statistical package for social sciences (SPSS) was used for data processing. Thus in the process of analysis, relationships or differences supporting or conflicting with original or new hypothesis were subjected to statistical test of significance to determine with what validity the data can be said to indicate any conclusions. All this material has been documented to have a coherent report comprising six sections.

Chapter one: Introduction gives the rationale behind the present research exercise. This section critically analyse different HIV Policies of the world, from North America to Europe to Africa to Asian Continent. It examine the existing HIV Policies, Programmes and Strategies

Chapter two: This chapter has been divided into three parts in order to fulfil the fourth objective "to study beneficiaries' perception of services rendered by Government and Non Governmental Organisations". The first part will discuss about the profile of the beneficiaries, the second part will discuss about their history on Drug use, Sexual and Medical History and their knowledge and risk perception on HIV/AIDS. The Third part will discuss about the beneficiaries perception on services provided by the Government and Non-Governmental Organisation.

Chapter three: This chapter has been divided into two parts to fulfil the second objective "to analyse the modalities of program implementation by the Government and Non-Governmental Organisations". First part will analyse the modalities of government program planning and implementation. The second part will deal with strategies and evaluations of ongoing program activities of Non Governmental organisation

Chapter four: In this chapter Non Governmental organisation will be subdivided into three sections a) Strategies and program activities of NGO's b) Role of social and cultural organisation c) Role of Faith Based Organisation. Social and Cultural organizations and Faith Based Organisations has been included as they play an important role in the prevention and mitigation of HIV and AIDS. India being a culturally diverse country, having strong cultural ethics, norms and values, it can go a long way in the prevention of HIV and AIDS by making use of these cultural organizations. Faith-based organizations are effective tools in responding to HIV and AIDS (Hogle, 2002).

Chapter five: This chapter discussed about Political commitment: Realities and Issues. Political commitment is a concept which is difficult to measure by a data which are collected routinely. Commitment is also multidimensional and therefore, cannot be measured through a single quantitative indicator. It might be possible to measure commitment directly if leaders were willing to submit to regular interviews about their level of understanding and support for HIV and AIDS programs. In order to find out commitment of the political leaders, a set of different questions were asked. Question ranges from policy making to program implementation and their involvement at the grassroots level taking into account not only the levels and degree of knowledge but also at the roots of the potential ignorance.

Chapter six: Recommendation and Conclusion chapter has been divided into six (6) Parts. The first part will fulfil the first objective: To study and examine the existing HIV Policies, Programmes and Strategies in Manipur and will be followed by conclusion and recommendation. Likewise the second part will fulfil the second objective: To analyze the modalities of program implementation by the Government and Non-Governmental Organisations. The third part will fulfil the third objective: To understand the political commitment of political leaders in HIV/AIDS mitigation. The fourth part will fulfil the fourth objective: To study beneficiaries perception of services rendered by Government and Non-Governmental Organisations. The fifth part will fulfil the fifth objective: To suggest the role of professional social workers in implementing prevention, care and support programmes in the field of HIV/AIDS and the corresponding conclusion and recommendation will follow. Finally the sixth part will give further scope of research in the topic.

CHAPTER 2

Profile of the Beneficiaries and their Opinions on the Services Availed

This chapter has been divided into three parts in order to fulfill the fourth objective “to study beneficiaries’ perception of services rendered by Government and Non Governmental Organisations”. The first part will discuss about the profile of the beneficiaries, the second part will discuss about their Personal history on Drug use, Sexual and Medical History and their knowledge and risk perception on HIV/AIDS. The Third part discuss about the beneficiaries perception on services provided by the Government and Non-Governmental Organisation.

The present study covering 12 Non-Governmental Organizations (NGOs) was conducted in and around Imphal east and west districts. These organizations were purposively selected, keeping in mind that they had been in existence for more than five years and were reaching out with the target groups with programs of HIV/AIDS mitigation. Further 5 beneficiaries were selected from each of the twelve organizations who were HIV positive.

PROFILES OF THE BENEFICIARIES

Age

It is well known that HIV infects people in the age group of 15 to 49 years; a population that is in the reproductive prime. Therefore age is an important factor in designing HIV intervention programmes.

The study highlighted that those who are using drugs and at the risk of contracting HIV/AIDS are in the age group of the most sexually active stage. The mean age for the present study is 33.5. The minimum age of the respondent is 24 and the maximum age is 50. The highest rate of HIV infection is in the age group of 31-40.

In the present study a sample of 60 respondents are taken into account in which all the respondents are HIV positive. Age is classified into three groups: 21-30, 31-40, 41-50. Among those who are infected with HIV, the age distribution pattern shows that a little more than half are in 31-40 years age group (see picture 2.1). The second most vulnerable groups are in the 21-30 age groups and only small percentage 8.33% are in the age group 41-50.

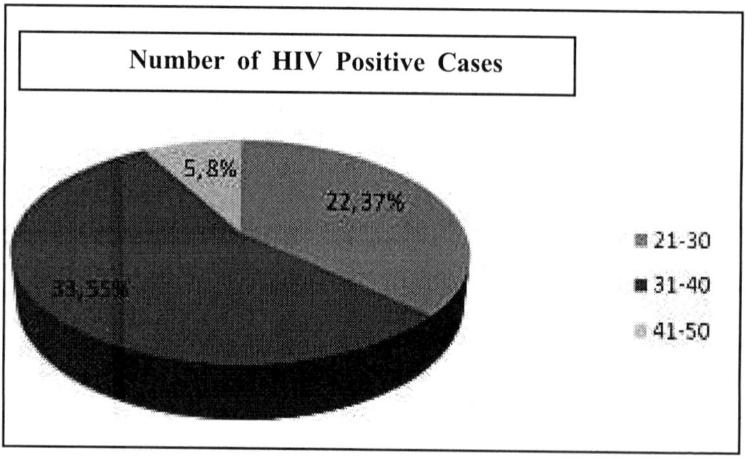

Fig. 2.1 Age group of Beneficiaries

Gender and Educational Level

In the prevention of HIV and AIDS infection, gender is a sensitive issue especially in the Indian context. Given the cultural context, often women are in a position where their vulnerability to HIV becomes higher, so also their power to negotiate for safer sex becomes weak. To add to these, talking about sex and sexuality is by and large a taboo.

In the present study, 60 respondents were interviewed using self designed semi structured interview Schedules. The gender distribution in the present study is given in Table 2.1 in which 66.67% of the respondents that is 40 were male respondents and the other 20 were female respondents. Male and female respondents are in the ratio of 2:1

Educational background

Education is the backbone of the society. Educations broaden the perspective of individuals and take rationale decision in life. Quite understandably, the educated are better off in the context of HIV and AIDS prevention (Jyoti K., 2005). In her study she further state that the rationale behind all programmes of AIDS prevention is generating awareness. Only when individuals become aware, would they self evaluate themselves as at risk and adopt protective behaviors.

The data in the present study shows that educational level of the respondents is not very high. As it can be seen on table 3.3 there is relationship between the level of education and the HIV positivity rate amongst the respondents. In the table 2.2 below it shows us that those whose education are till secondary has the highest number of HIV positivity rate 41.67%.

People who studied up to secondary level has positivity rate of 41% and the second highest 23% is in the group of respondents who studied up to graduation level. The higher the level of education is the lower the rate of HIV positivity. Educating and giving in-depth knowledge about HIV prevention to those who are at high risk of HIV infection would yield the most desirable outcome.

Table 2.1 Cross Tabulation on Gender and Educational Level

		Educational Level					Total
		Primary	Secondary	Hr. Secondary	Graduate	Post Graduate	
Gender	Male	3	18	7	11	1	40
	female	4	7	6	3	0	20
Total		7	25	13	14	1	60

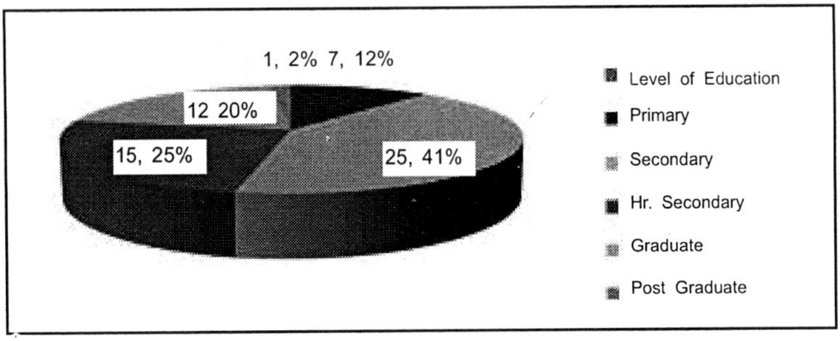

Fig. 2.2 Relationships between level of education and HIV positivity

The above given argument could be supported by a similar study conducted by Singh H., et al 2010, among 90 HIV positive tribal patients in Chhattisgarh in which the result shows us that low level of education among the people aggravates the risk of HIV infection. They conclude that there was a high frequency of behavioral risk factors, together with unawareness, and very little health infrastructure, thus creating an impending risk for the rapid spread of HIV and AIDS.

Language

It is well known that language is an important forms of communication by which human beings can interact, share their views and thoughts. It is known that there are thousands of languages and dialects in which human beings communicate. In the context of HIV/AIDS it is important that the communicator reaches the target audience.

Communication is the process of conveying information from a sender to a receiver with the use of a medium in which the communicated information is understood the same way by both the sender and the receiver. It is a process that allows the sender and the receiver to exchange information by several methods. It is important that the one who communicates reaches the target audience in the right way how he wanted to transfer his information's especially in the case of HIV/AIDS preventions. Communication is defined as a process by which we assign and convey meaning in an attempt to create shared understanding. This process requires a vast repertoire of skills in intrapersonal and interpersonal processing, listening, observing, speaking, questioning, analyzing, and evaluating.

The language and dialects spoken in the study area includes Manipuri and different dialects of the state. According to census of India 2001 in Manipur there are 32 different distinct dialects spoken by distinct tribes of the state.

Out of the total respondents n=60, 81.7% of the respondents spoke Manipuri dialect and 18.3 % spoke tribal dialects.

Marital Status

Needless to state, detection of HIV in one family member can throw the entire family in turmoil. Media has often highlighted travails of women who were thrown out once found tested HIV positive. On the other hand there are instances where HIV negative spouse has offered unconditional support and care to the infected partner. Definitely multiple factors interact to determine how a family response to HIV. The situation of those who are single or unmarried for different reasons is not much better. Instead of taking care of their parents the situation becomes reversed. Elders of a family often have to carry the burden of the disease.

Sexual behavior patterns are different for different age groups as the ages of the respondents in the present study are in the most sexually active groups. There are gender differences in sexual behavior patterns among men and women. Understanding these differences is important to plan gender based intervention strategies in order to ensure that people living with HIV have a better quality of life, addressing their sexual concerns both within and outside of the marriage.

Table 2.2 shows us that out of the total respondents 43.33% of them are single, 56.67% are married where 38.33% living with spouse and 15% of the respondents are married and divorced/ separated respectively. Majority of the respondents pick up the habit of drug use before their marriage. Drug use and sharing of needles and syringes were a culture during the 80's, which is also the main reason for the routes of HIV transmission in the state.

Table 2.2 Cross Tabulation of Gender and Marital status

Gender	Marital Status				Total
	Single	married	divorced/ seperated	any other	
Male	24	12	4	0	40
Female	2	11	5	2	20
Total	26	23	9	2	60

HIV status and actual age of marriage

Among the 60 respondents, the mean age of marriage is 25.38. During the study, it was discovered that there were few respondents who are well aware of their serostatus, but got married after mutual consent by both the partners. In one such incident a case of ** Ms Sonia and *Mr. Jiten a couple who are both HIV positive and are working together in the same organization. They came in contact with each other through an NGO where they are presently working. In due course of time they became closer. They shared each other's problem and one day they finally decided to tie the knot. It was a mutual understanding between them, both taking into consideration the pros and cons of marriage as they are both HIV positive. They consulted their parents and finally got married, worked together and lived happily until the time of interview. * Ms Sonia and *Mr. Jiten name changed to protect identity.* The mean age of the spouse is 31.52 with the minimum of 16 and maximum age of the spouse 64. The mean number of years married is 8.78 years. The minimum number of years the respondents are married is 2years and the maximum is 22. Among the respondents, there are HIV positive couples who properly monitor and maintain their health. These types of people are longer married and lived a healthy life as compared to others who do not maintain their health.

Family and Number of children

Majority of the respondents are from nuclear family, only 1.66% of the respondents are from joint family. The mean number of children one has is 2.38. The minimum number of children one has is 1 and the maximum is 8. Among the respondents 28 have children and the majority of the respondents have 1 or 2 child only. 42.85% has 2 children followed by 35.71% have 1 child only.

Employment and nature of employment

The HIV/AIDS pandemic has affected almost every aspect of people's lives and has created problems of discrimination, loss of dignity and lack of privacy for people living with HIV/AIDS. The pandemic also tends to create a fear psychosis, anxiety among the general populace, which leads to a mixed response. In the employment sector, companies, individuals and organizations responded differently to the epidemic utilizing various strategies and in the absence of laws and policies to guide these various agencies, there is a real danger that human rights are compromised.

Figure 2.3 shows that out of the total beneficiaries who are employed, maximum of them are self employed with 30%. Negligible numbers are employed in the government sector, NGO's and Services.

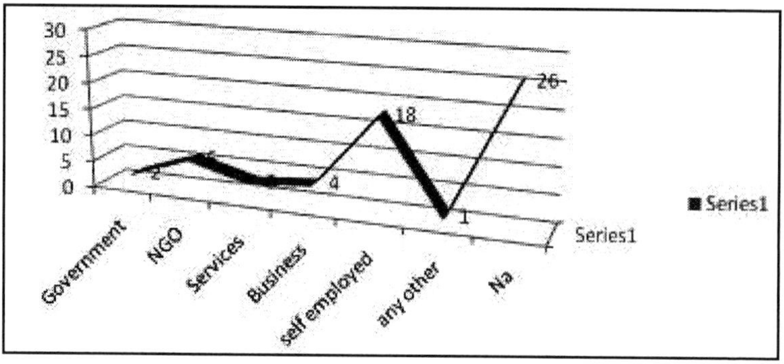

Fig. 2.3 Nature of Employment

Income and Savings if any

As the AIDS pandemic enters into its third decade, it is hitting particularly hard in communities in poor states and urban communities who has a higher rates of unemployment, poor housing, poor health, early death due to poor infrastructure on health facilities.

The respondent have a mean salary of Rs. 4186.67/- with minimum salary of Rs. 1500/- and maximum salary of Rs. 8000/-. Incomes of the respondents, families and spouse taken together n=60 have a mean salary of Rs. 6866.67/- with minimum salary of Rs. 6000/ - and maximum salary of Rs. 15000/-. Among the beneficiaries not a single respondent could save a part of their earnings as they have to cough up with the rising prices whether in medicos or in their daily needs.

PERSONAL HISTORY

Personal history of the beneficiaries has been divided into four parts. It is important to understand and know about the personal history of the beneficiaries as this would be instrumental in analysis on how they have been infected or affected. First part is about understanding the knowledge level of the beneficiaries on HIV/ AIDS and their risk perception on it. Second part will look into history their Drug use and linkages to HIV/AIDS. Thirdly it will discuss about sexual history and finally on their medical history.

HIV and STI Knowledge

Knowledge and understanding about the subject or a particular thing makes a person aware of the facts and the consequences of it and they act accordingly. Knowledge according to Oxford English Dictionary is the acquisition of expertise and skills through experience or education; the theoretical or practical understanding of a subject; what is known in a particular field or in total; facts and information and awareness or familiarity gained by experience of a fact or situation. Knowledge acquisition involves complex cognitive processes: perception, learning, communication, association and reasoning.

The knowledge and awareness level on HIV/AIDS and related infectious diseases differs from one individual to another. Knowledge level of each individual differs from one another. Out of the total respondent of n=60 every respondents are aware of HIV and AIDS. It wouldn't be an exaggeration to say that most of the respondents are aware of HIV and AIDS if not there is in-depth knowledge about its complexities.

Apart from HIV and AIDS there is various illness or diseases which are inter twined together. Cases can be cited of Tuberculosis, Hepatitis and Sexually Transmitted Infections where they play a host pathogen for the HIV to enter human body in various ways. Of the many respondents, their knowledge levels on Tuberculosis, Hepatitis and Sexually Transmitted Diseases are good. It can be concluded that many of the respondents are aware about the said infections

Knowledge level on the technicalities and the how and why of HIV infections also varies amongst the respondents. Out of the many ways of HIV infections five choices were given to the respondents' viz Unprotected sexual intercourse, use of infected Needles and Syringes, Infected blood transfusion, from infected mother to child and all the above sources.

Table 2.3 Knowledge level on various modes of HIV transmission

Various Modes of HIV Transmission	Frequency	Percent
unprotected sexual intercourse	2	3.3
infected needles and syringes	1	1.7
infected blood transfusion	1	1.7
from infected mother to child	1	1.7
all the above	55	91.7
Total	60	100.0

A total of n=60 respondents answered to the question. A total of 55 respondents which forms 91.7% are well aware of the four main routes of HIV infection, while other respondents comprising 1.7% each of the total respondent gave the reason from infected mother to child, sharing infected Needles & Syringes and Infected blood transfusion. Also 3.3% gave answer to unprotected sexual intercourse.

Risk Perceptions and Discrimination

Risk perception is the subjective assessment of the probability of a specified type of accident happening and how concerned we are with the consequences. To perceive risk includes evaluations of the probability as well as the consequences of a negative outcome. It may also be argued that as affects related to the activity is an element of risk perception. It could also be said that it is an unrealistic optimism or illusion of control about future events. Perception of risk goes beyond the individual, and it is a social and cultural construct reflecting values, symbols, history, and ideology (Weinstein, N.D., 1980).

Similar cases of discrimination and fear of disclosure prevails among the women respondents in the present study. * *Ms Mala age 32 is a widow HIV positive patient who has been married to an IDU for almost 14 years. Ms Mala got married to*Mr. Chaoba at the prime of her age. Both the spouse was doing fine until one day when her in-laws discovered that their son is an HIV positive patient. They blame their daughter in-law to be the carrier of the disease which she passed on to their son. They started neglecting her, pick up unnecessary arguments. Life was even miserable to her when her husband expired. Being uneducated and not getting financial or material support from her in-laws, Ms Mala was forced to go back to her parental home. Until the time of this personal interview she joined a group of positive people and worked with an NGO as a peer educator. *Ms Mala and Mr. Chaoba name changed to protect identity.*

Table 2.4 is self explanatory. A total of 20% of the respondents felt a sense of discrimination by the officials and staffs at the ART centre. But contrary to the negative sense of discrimination there are 20% of the respondents who felt the officials and the staff are co-operative. Many of the respondents also felt that staff and officials are slowly co-operating. If given in the form of percentages 23.3% each of the respondents are of the opinion that they felt a sense of discrimination in the past but staffs are more cooperative now and drugs are available on time unless the two national highways are blocked.

Most of the respondents in the study groups face discrimination from various quarters. A total of 60% among the respondents of n=36 face discrimination from the society. The other 11.7% faces discrimination from families and in-laws.

Table 2.4 Experience at the ART centre

Particulars of problems at the ART Centre	Frequency	%age
Personnel's are cooperative	12	20
Felt a sense of discrimination by the official & staff	12	20
Forgetting the past they are cooperative now	14	23.3
Drugs are available on time	14	23.3
Travelling is a problem	5	8.4
Priorities given to known people	3	5
any other		
Total	60	100

Majority of the respondents complained the in appropriate support structures in their communities and societies. A total of 41.7% faces discrimination of various types from the communities. Most of them complain of receiving a comments from the communities, not allowing them to participate in community events, not allowing them in community self help groups etc.

During an informal conversation to office staffs during the study period; many of the people do not perceive that they are at risk of infections. They consider people will have infections only if they are involved in an activity as described to be the means of HIV infection. Acceptance level and awareness on HIV and AIDS thus increased manifold but people still lack in-depth knowledge of HIV and AIDS.

A great majority of the respondents were willing to help with AIDS education in the study area. More than half of respondents were willing to care for relatives if they were infected with HIV. However, also about half of the study population believes that people with HIV/AIDS should be identified and isolated from the community. Almost half of the study population was worried about becoming infected with HIV, but only 7% were aware of their own personal vulnerability. Students were the most concerned about the threat of AIDS. According to study conducted by Thomas J., et al 1999 Most respondents in the study groups are generally aware of how HIV/AIDS is transmitted and supported HIV/AIDS, sex, and drug education in schools. 76% believed AIDS education could reduce the transmission of HIV among young people.

Though many of the respondents are well aware of HIV infection in the study group their perception on risk differs with each individual. According to study conducted by Lee, T., et al 2006 among Injecting Heroin users in Taiwan all respondents had adequate knowledge about HIV/AIDS, but held misconceptions regarding the modes of HIV transmission. They concluded that many respondents who did not perceived themselves susceptible to AIDS rarely use condoms and occasionally shared needles.

In the present study 48.3% of the respondents are in the habit of drinking Alcohol and drug use. It can be said that under the influence of Alcohol and drugs people tends to get involved in a risky behavior which the respondents doesn't necessarily perceived it to be risky.

The general perceptions, beliefs, knowledge, behavior and attitudes of the respondent differ according to their level of education in the present study group. Those with higher educational level fair better than those with lower level of education. During an informal interaction during the study period with the nursing staff and Doctor's of a government hospital in Manipur, what one perceived and the reality are wide apart. There are hundreds of Doctors who are being trained by the state government in Manipur in the areas of HIV and AIDS. But only a handful of them really practice it, giving a reason of what they perceived to be a risky job to help fight the diseases.

A personal visit to the Integrated Counseling and Testing Centre's (ICTC) and observing the client flow patterns and HIV test uptake tells a different story altogether. In one of the testing centre there was no maintenance of confidentiality. Clients who are being advised by someone for HIV testing are made seated in the same room while simultaneous counseling of other client is going on.

There are no separate counselors for men, women and children. In one of the worst case scenario where *Mr. Pankaj* went to a T.B Hospital for check up, he was also advised to go for HIV* *testing. He then goes to government owned ICTC's centre in the heart of the capital. The normal procedure for HIV testing is to conduct pre-test counseling, advising them of the many possible outcomes. His blood sample was drawn for the necessary testing. He was called again to collect the test outcome after few days. The test result shows non reactive. Had it been the reverse side of it, what would become of him as he was also not given post test counseling? Mr. Pankaj himself took initiative and went to enquire again after learning that pre-test and post test counseling is a must in HIV testing. He enquired about the lack of counseling and the reply to it was insufficient counselors to handle the job. * Mr. Pankaj name changed to protect Identity.*

A study conducted by Joseph S., et al 2010, on sex differentials in the uptake of HIV testing shows that men's and women's testing patterns are not consistent. They made a community-based, cross-sectional survey among 347 people living with HIV in three HIV high prevalence districts of India and examined their reason for undergoing an HIV test. They say that men were more likely to be advised to test by a private practitioner and to test in the private sector. Women were more likely to be advised to test by a family member, and to test in the public sector. Men were more likely to receive pre-test information than women, when tested in the private sector. Men were also more likely to receive direct disclosure of their HIV positive status by a health provider, regardless of the sector in which they tested. More women than men were repeatedly tested for HIV, regardless of sector. They concluded that examining gender dynamics that underpin sex differentials in HIV testing patterns and practices is essential for a realistic assessment of the challenges and implications of scaling-up HIV testing and mainstreaming gender in HIV/AIDS programmes.

Drug Use History

Drug use during the later part of the 20th century in the north east and Manipur in particular was a culture. People from various backgrounds were trapped in the habit of drug use. Drugs were easily available through the porous border of Moreh an International border of India and the then Burma (Myanmar). Myanmar was considered the drug capital of the south East Asia as also it lies in the notorious golden triangle where heroin was produced, locally known as No. 4. According to findings by Rafiey H., et al 2009 needle and syringe sharing has increased among female injection drug users in Iran especially those who are being jobless, having illegal income, drug use by family members. They identified that drug use for enjoyment and peer pressure as causes of first injection, first injection in roofless and roofed public places. They usually inject at the groin area, injection at scrotum and they have lifetime experience of nonfatal overdose and history of arrest in the past years.

Age at onset of drug use (oral/Injection)

The mean age of oral drug use among the respondents was 20.56 and the mean age of Injection drug use was 23.59. The respondents started using of oral drugs as early as 15 years and goes up to 29. Whereas the youngest injection drug users were 17 and some even started injecting at the later age of 37.

Types of drugs

The different types of drugs used by the respondents are Heroin, Diazepam, Spasmo Proxivon, Marijuana, Nitrovite tablets, Cough Syrups, Adhesive solution, Brown sugar, Tidigesic, Calmpose, Buprenorphine, Alcohol and Alprazolam, etc. The most commonly used drugs by the respondents are Heroin 91.2%, Diazepam 40%, Spasmo proxivon 72.5%, Marijuana 55%, Nitrovite tablets 47.5%, cough syrups 47.5%, Adhesive solution 27.5%, Buprenorphine 22.5%, Alcohol 65%. The above percentages are calculated on the basis of 60 respondents and taking above 5% of particular drugs they are using. Most of the respondents are using more than one drug during their lifetime.

Frequency of drug use on a daily basis

It was found that most of the respondents use drugs more than once in a day. 45% of the respondents' uses thrice in a day, 32.5% use four times in a day, 15% use twice in a day. 2.5% only once and 2.5% above four times in a day. Another 5% use drugs as when they have money to get the stuff.

Nature of drug use (alone/Company) equipment sharing/not sharing past and present

The study reveals that those who are addicted to drug use, they usually take in the company of friends. It was more of a culture during the days to get together on a particular spot and share their drugs. Only 15% of the respondents are using drugs alone without the company of friends. The rest 85% of the respondents use drugs in the company of friends. In the past 90% of the respondents shares their equipment of drug injection. Only 10% of the respondents do not share their injection equipment in the past. 97.5% of the present users do not share their injection equipment. 2.5% of the present users do not share their Gun (Syringes- local terminology) but they share their other equipments like distilled water for mixing with drugs, containers, etc.

Abstinence

A total of 71.8% of the respondents at least once gave up using of drugs even if it is for a day or so. Another 50% of the respondents gave up using of drugs for more than 6 weeks.13.3% each gave up for 4 to 6 days and 6 days to 2 weeks. 10% gave up for 2 to 4 days only, 6.7% gave up for 4 to 6 weeks and 3.3% each gave up for 0 to 2 days and 2 weeks to 4 weeks. The cases of relapse are also high among the drug users. More than 50% of the respondents have relapse cases. 86.7% of the relapse cases are due to peer pressure, 6.7% contribute due to anger and 3.3% each complained due to loss of job and depression. 48.3% of the total respondents have atleast once been admitted to de-addiction centre/ rehabilitation centre. 33.3% have been there 2 times, 13.3% of the respondents have been to the centre 3 times and 26.7% each have gone through 1 times and more than four times respectively.

Drug use and HIV linkage

It is learnt from study conducted by Kheirandish P., et al 2010, that incarceration increases the chances of HIV infection among inmates of prison. It is a well known fact that Manipur is famous for its popularity in various co-curricular activities like sports in India and internationally. It is also not less popular in drug use as the first cases of HIV infection was detected in the blood samples collected from Injecting Drug users in the state. Drug use among the people was popular during the later part of 1980's. Drug use, police commandoes, imprisonment, lodging in prison and taking bribe by the police was the watch word of the state during the time.

Before the implementation of the drug substitution programme in the state, there were many difficulties faced by the government in cracking down drug peddlers and drug users. But after the implementation of the drug substation therapy and the programme taken up by many renowned NGO's many of the drug users came up, share their problems and tackling the problem takes a new shape.

In spite of the initiatives taken up by the governmental and nongovernmental organization, the number of drug users being caught by the police and being detained or not detained didn't decrease.

Table 2.5 shows us that among the total respondents there are 58.33% which form 35 of the total respondents were at least once caught by police because of their drug use. The other respondent 7 which form 11.67% of the respondents had never been caught by the police. The rate of detention in correspond to the number caught didn't match according to the findings. In the present study 58.33% were caught and only 6.7% of them are in the lock up or jail.

Table 2.5 Percentage of respondents ever been caught by the police

Response	Frequency	Percent
Yes	35	58.33%
No	7	11.67%
NA	18	30%
Total n=60	60	100%

When interacted with those people who are being caught, they say that they are being let off the hook if they have money to pay to the police personnel. The other 6.7% of the respondents said that they were not in handy with money at the time they were caught, so they have to spend the night at the police lock up. The next day their family members would be informed and they would be bailed out.

The brighter side of the police story shows that during the earlier year's people who are being caught by the police are lodged in the police lock up for the night and they are sent to Jail. But the present day's police are aware of the human rights activities so they never sent drug users to prison. The other reason could be that the prison capacity does not allow them to do so as one of the respondents said during interaction. He further said that they use to inject drugs inside the jail premises during the earlier years by sharing Needles and Syringes. They procure their drugs through jail staff by selling their belongings like Jewellery, Jackets, watches etc.

There are various sources of funds from which the drug users procure their drugs inside the jail premises. It ranges from families, friends and relatives and to the extent of selling their own belongings. Out of the total respondents only one respondent use drugs inside the jail premises and he got the funds from families and relatives. Of the respondent who uses drugs inside the jail he said that he got it from his peers and colleagues.

Many of the respondent hints the importance of introducing awareness programs inside the jail premises. A total of 23 respondents felt the need to introduce awareness generation program inside the jail premises.

The components of awareness programs which can be introduced in the jail premises are categorized into

1) legal rights
2) Information Education and Communication
3) Treatment
4) care and support
5) after care

6) any other

7) NA/DK.

A total of n=21 respondents answered to the questions on what are the components of awareness programmes they would like it to be introduced inside the jail premises. Each respondents were given the choice of answering three multiple answers. A total of n=17 respondents would like to see that legal rights awareness be introduced inside the jail premises. Those respondents cited the reason behind their choices, that out of their experiences they saw many of the people especially those inside the jail are not aware of their basic rights. Then n=8 respondents would like to see Information Education and Communication programmes on HIV and AIDS be introduced inside the jail premises, so that the authorities and the inmates are well aware of the nitty-gritty of the HIV pandemic.

As far as Treatment is concerned n=13 respondents would like to see that it is introduced inside the jail premises. Most of the respondents are aware that some PLHA are inside the jail, so they wanted that adherence to treatment practices and the various knowledge of treatment should be made known to the authorities. As everyone knows that substance abuse complicates both HIV/AIDS and its management because of the effects that illicit drugs have on various body systems and the behavioral disturbances that accompany substance use. For a variety of reason, adherence to treatment is poor in this population and several factors have a negative impact on adherence. Treatment of drug abusers who are HIV-positive requires more flexibility than treating drug abuse and HIV separately. Because medication regimens can be complicated and demanding and non adherence to treatment can cause mutation of the virus resulting in drug-resistant strains, it is essential to get the patient committed to treatment. It is important that proper treatment regiment is made known to the jail authorities.

In the case of care and support programmes to be introduced inside the jail premises n=19 respondents gave their consent over it. As we all know Care and support play a critical role in assisting people who are HIV-positive to understand the need for prevention and to enable them to protect others. As the HIV/AIDS pandemic progresses and HIV-seropositive individuals contend with devastating illness, timely help and support from family and other authorities is vital in the control of HIV infections.

After care and support services are being extended to the people, it is vital that a follow up services to the clients are properly maintained.

Sexual History

The most common forms of HIV transmission in Manipur was due to sharing of contaminated Needles and Syringes during the earlier days. But now the trend of HIV infection has been shifted to the general population through sexual routes. According to Van Dam C.J 1994 sexual intercourse is the most important mode of HIV spread globally. He said that according to accumulated evidence there is a relationship between STI and HIV infection in threefold ways: the presence of an STI is a mark of risk behavior for HIV infection, STIs are biological cofactors for HIV transmission, and concurrent HIV infection increases the virulence of some STI pathogens. Unprotected sexual intercourse with multiple partners predisposes one to HIV infection.

The incidence of both HIV infection and other STIs therefore indicates the practice of high risk sex behavior in a community. He also said that increased incidence of HIV infection has been found in people with genital ulcer disease. It is therefore likely that genital ulcerations caused by traditional STIs provide easy entry or exit points for HIV.

According to Cicely M., et al 2006, young people assess potential sexual partners as “clean” or “unclean”; sexual partners have an important influence on behavior. Condoms are stigmatizing and associated with lack of trust; gender stereotypes are crucial in determining social expectations and, in turn, behavior. There are penalties and rewards for sex from society; reputations and social displays of sexual activity or inactivity are important; and social expectations hamper communication about sex. They conclude that young people who are involved in unprotected sexual intercourse have higher chances of HIV infection than those who are not.

Table 2.6 represents the age of the respondents when they first experience sexual initiation. The age group is divided into three categories ages 15-20, 21-25 and 26-30. The age group 21-25 represents the most sexually active group among the respondents comprising 45% of the total respondents. The second highest group is 15-20 and form 16.67% of the total respondents. The table can be interpreted that young boys and girls who are most sexually active have a higher risk of HIV infection.

Table 2.6 Age at when sexual initiation experienced

Age group	Frequency	percentage
15-20	10	16.67%
21-25	27	45%
26-30	2	3.33%
NA	21	35%
Total	60	100%

Particular question on the frequency of condom used and the reasons were asked among the respondents. It can be seen that out of the total respondents 25% uses every time they had sexual intercourse, 5% says they usually use quite often, 8.33% says they use sometimes when it is readily available. Although condoms are available in many of the departmental stores and pharmacies, the above data's shows that it is not really within the reach of the clients every time.

The reason given by the respondents were categorized into four groups, to avoid pregnancy, protect self and partner from STI and HIV/AIDS, both to avoid pregnancy and to protect self and partner s from STI and HIV/AIDS and any other. A total of 4.17% uses condom to avoid pregnancy, 12.5% use it to protect self and partner from STI and HIV/AIDS, 83.33% use it to protect both from pregnancy and self and partner from STI and HIV/AIDS. A total of six respondents gave reason for not using the condom and the rest 54 respondents don't respond to the question. 1.67% of the respondents says they don't use condom because it reduces sexual pleasure and another 8.33% gave one or more reasons like non availability on time, trust within the sexual partners etc.

Sexual relationship between the respondents and commercial sex workers (CSW) were studied among 60 respondents. Out of the total n=60, 16.7% of the total says they have visited and had sexual experience with the commercial sex workers during their past life. A total of 83.3% replies in the negative. Another 1.7% of the total respondents reply in the affirmative that they are currently visiting the commercial sex workers. The frequency of visits were taken among the sample and 10% says that they visited the CSW more than four times in a month and the other 3.33% each visited once and twice respectively. Out of the total respondents 8.33% uses every time they visited the CSW's, 1.67% use it quite often and another 3.33% use it when it is available.

Medical History

Health is the most important assets of any individual. Among the present study group of n=60 beneficiaries they are all HIV positive. As described earlier Manipur is a landlocked area which lies in the extreme north eastern states of India bordering Myanmar by 358 km sq. Due to communication problem especially road transportation, medical aid and other essential commodities are not available on time. When medical aid is not available on time the poor communities are the hardest hit especially those who are HIV positive. People living with HIV and AIDS has to shell out their hard earned money to buy food for daily use in an exorbitant rates comparing to the maximum price printed on the items. They are then left with no money to buy nutritional support as they are taking daily dose of ART. Naturally they are bound to be in a deteriorating health conditions. Out of the total 60 respondents 98.3% has answered to the question on whether they have had cough or fever during the past six months. 58.3% said yes and 40.7% said no to the question. Of the respondents who have answered yes 40% had cough or fever lasting for 2 to 4 days. 34.28% had cough or fever lasting for 4 days to 1 week. 17.14% had for more than 2 weeks, followed by 2.91% for 0 to 2 days and 8.6% for 1week to 2 weeks. In respect to consultation of medical professionals 30% met registered medical practitioner for consultation, 10% use home remedy, 6.7% goes for self medication and 5% refer to private medical practitioner. A total of 60 respondents which forms 100% of the total respondents answered yes to the question on whether they have undergone any diagnostic investigation during the last three years. Rising price on medical aid and other essential commodities has had an adverse health impact on the people living with HIV and AIDS. Poor PLHA people cannot afford to private medical aid and they are forced to remain as they are whatever the health conditions might be.

Out of the total respondents n=60 in the table 2.7 shows that the ratio of male and female who goes for blood testing is 40:20. A gender difference in the uptake of HIV testing shows that men and women testing patterns are not consistent. (Joseph S., et al 2010).

Table 2.7 percentage of male and female who goes for blood investigation

Gender	Blood investigation Yes	Percentage
male	40	66.67%
female	20	33.33%
Total	60	100%

The percentage of those who goes for blood testing clearly indicates that there is a sex differential in the uptake of HIV testing in the state. As stated earlier when interacted with women respondents of the state in the present study group, they are reluctant to go for blood testing due to various reasons. They have heard of many stories about discrimination of the womenfolk especially of those who are married to IDU's. Out of n=60 only 33.33% of the women respondents goes for blood testing against 66.67% of their male counterpart. They feared of being detected HIV positive since their husbands are ex drug users and moreover they are feared of being turned away by their in-laws.

One women of such cases narrates her story, *Ms Shanti* 37 years of age was married to her school boyfriend Mr. Thoiba* when she was only 19 years old. Her boyfriend was frequented to* *parties and functions organized by the community. He was also a rock singer quite popular among her friends in school. The first reason she said she was attracted to him was due to his popularity among her friends. She never knew he was into drugs at the beginning.*

As time goes by they are more familiar with each other and the intensity for their love grew even stronger. They go together for birthday parties, kitty parties, song concerts and other get together parties like picnics, marriages etc.

When both of them graduated together from college they plan to get married. They finally walk the Aisle together and *shared their marriage vow. They were happily married until one day when she discovered the he was injecting drugs inside their room while she was preparing food. They were living together with her husband family. Day by day he increases the frequency of his shots (Injecting Drugs), then his health condition worsened. Fear of being discovered they kept together as a secret. Finally when his condition can no more be kept secret, the consequence response was his death. Before his death some of his friend advised him to go for a medical checkup and his blood test result for HIV was reactive. It was too late to react or go for medication. His parents didn't exactly knows the reason for his death as the Doctor told them that it was a case of multiple heart failure, Jaundice and T.B. She was the only one who was informed of his HIV status. Then she was also advised by the Doctor to get HIV test done, where the result proved to be reactive.

She narrated; she was afraid of declaring her condition to her in-laws as she knew some of her friends being turn away by their in-laws. She was left with two kids to be taken care of. She now works in one of the nongovernmental organization and supports her kids. . * Ms Shanti and Mr. Thoiba name changed to protect identity

The above case study shows that there would be many women like her who are not aware of their sero-status or who don't want to disclose their sero-status. It would not be an exaggeration to say that there are high probabilities of womenfolk's whose health conditions are not properly taken care of due to their sero-status.

Table 2.8 Percentage of male and female who are HIV positive

Gender	Frequency yes	Percentage
male	40	40
female	20	20
Total	60	60

Table 2.8 shows that among the respondent of n=60 there are 20 women and 40 men who goes for blood testing and all the 20 women and 40 men are diagnosed HIV positive. The exact rate of positivity cannot be either concluded and say that positivity rates are higher among women who got tested for HIV infection or their men counterpart. Whatever the case may be it can be said that the health condition of the womenfolk of the state are worse than their male counterpart. In general, majority of the respondents are from socially- economically backward classes. Women of the state enjoy almost equal status with their male counterpart of the state and they also constitute the workforce of the state. The respondent's low economic status forces them to work in unorganized sectors. They are mostly vegetable vendors, run Pan Shop (Beetel Nut Shop) and other minor jobs. So when their health condition worsened their livelihoods are being cut of as they don't have other means of income.

OPINION ON SERVICES AVAILED BY BENEFICIARIES FROM GO,S AND NGO,S

The government through its various organizations and departments provide a wide variety of services to the beneficiaries. Some of the main services provided by the government are 1) counseling services 2) referral services 3) clinical test for HIV and other contagious diseases 4) treatment and prevention services, etc. Apart from the above listed services provided by the government the nongovernment organization also provides detoxification services for drug users and Needle and syringe exchange services.

Table 2.9 below a total of n= 60 respondents were asked on the services they received from the government. Each respondent were given the right to give multiple answers up to 3 choices. Since the respondents can give three answers of their choice the total frequency will be more than the total number of respondents and the corresponding frequencies. A total of 95% respondents said they received services like clinical test for HIV and other STI test. Most of the government and NGO centre's provide counseling services, 91.67% of the total respondents said they received counseling services. Certain cases under unavoidable circumstance or when particular services are sought by the beneficiaries they are being referred to NGO or Care home by the government. Of the total respondents 33.33% were referred to care homes or NGO's for specific services. As far as treatment and prevention services are concerned 78.33% enjoyed the services from the government.

Table 2.9 Services provided by the government

Services	Frequency	Percent
Counseling	55	91.67%
referral services	20	33.33%
clinical test	57	95%
treatment & prevention services	47	78.33%

Table 2.10 below, respondents were given the right to choose three answers of their choice. Due to possibility of multiple answers the total frequency will exceeds the total respondents and the corresponding percentages can be greater than 100. Out of the total respondents of n=60, 75% of the total respondents received counseling services through NGOs. Majority of the NGO's used referral services as many of the NGOs are interlinked together. Of the total respondents 55% received referral services.

There are hardly any NGO's which provide clinical test facilities for STI, HIV etc. In the present study none of the respondents received testing facilities from the nongovernmental organizations. Treatment, prevention and after care services are very popular among the different NGO's working in the field of HIV and AIDS. Out of the total respondents n=60, 40% of the respondents received the said services.

Table 2.10 Services provided by the Non Governmental Organizations

Services	Frequency	Percent
counseling	45	75%
Referral Services	33	55%
treatment & prevention services	24	40%
detoxification for drug use	37	61.67%
needle and syringe exchange program	36	60%
all of the above	4	6.67%

Manipur is well known for the fact that the first HIV was detected among the blood samples collected from intravenous drug users. Since then the government of Manipur in collaboration with various ministries of the central government and help from various international organization started HIV and AIDS intervention programs. Taking examples from various successful stories from the globe, the Government of Manipur started Rapid Intervention and Care projects (RIAC) under Manipur State AIDS control Society. The main objective of the RIAC project was to halt and reverse the HIV pandemic among the Intravenous Drug Users. Drug detoxification program takes a new shape and was very successful in the context of Manipur as the presence of HIV among Intravenous drug users came down drastically after the inception of the program.

Out of the total respondents of n=60, 61.67% utilized the services of drug detoxification services being provided by the nongovernmental organization. The process and strategy followed by many of the nongovernmental organization varies according to time, place, location and community. Some of the most common strategy being followed by these organizations is detoxification for a period lasting for 5 days. During this period, clients are assessed and proper strategy is carried out to suit the particular client's needs and taking into consideration the gravity of his addictions. Then each client is given a proper dose of drugs and the doses are reduced on a routine basis.

Needle and Syringe Exchange Program (NSEP) is a big hit among the NGO's who are working on Intravenous drug users. Various research studies on Needle and Syringe exchange program around the globe shows that it is a big success in the prevention of HIV and AIDS. Among the total respondents of n=60, 60% of the respondents enjoyed this services. In spite of the success in NSEP there are many difficulties in the implementation. When interacted with the respondents who are receiving NSEP services in the NGO's they have many complaints about the program. Many of the respondents complained that the law enforcing agencies sometimes harassed them, when they carry used Syringes. In NSEP, clients are required to submit the used Syringes in exchange for the fresh ones. Many clients say that, the law enforcing agencies are taking advantage of people who carry used Syringes and charge them some money in order to avoid unnecessary detention.

A total respondents of n=60 were asked whether they received Needles and Syringes regularly from the NGO's. Majority of the respondents n=50 which forms 83.33% of the total respondents say they receive it regularly. As far as ART is concern a total of n=60 were asked on whether they receive ART regularly from the government, 100% say they received it regularly.

A total of n=60 respondents were asked on whether they have ever heard of National AIDS Control Program Phase III and IV. The details given in Table 2.11 shows that 100% of the total respondents have heard about NACP III and IV.

Table 2.11 Awareness about NACP III &IV

Response	Frequency	Percent
Yes	60	100.0

A total of n=60 respondents were asked on whether they have ever heard of National AIDS Control Program Phase III and IV. The details given in Table 2.11 shows that 100% of the total respondents have heard about NACP III and IV.

A total of n=60 respondents were asked on their understanding about the various components of NACP III. The level of understanding were categorized into a) Very Good b) Good c) Fair d) Any other and NA/DK

In Table 2.12, the percentage level of understanding about the different components of NACP III is clearly given. Out of the total respondents 81.7% say that their level of understanding about prevention (T.I, STI Care, ICTC, Blood Safety, IEC, Condom promotion) is good and 18.3% says that their level of understanding is fair.

As far as Care (Treatment of O.I, Provision of free DOT treatments, PEP, ART) is concern 28.3% and 71.7% says that their level of understanding is good and fair respectively.

Partnership and collaboration is the most important components of HIV and AIDS prevention. As we all know HIV/AIDS has no boundary irrespective of class, caste, religion and rich or poor. It affects each one individual in one way or the other. So when it comes to prevention intervention, every individual has a part or role to play. The government should also involve different ministries like education, sports, health, tourism etc. in order to effectively control the spread of the diseases. Knowing of the importance, a total respondents of n=60 were asked on their understanding about Collaboration (GIPA, Inter sectoral collaboration, Involvement of ministries, workplace intervention etc.). A total of 11.7% and 88.3% of the respondents say that their understanding about collaboration is good and fair respectively.

Capacity building and timely training of the staff and personnel's are important for the programme to be successful. Also if a programme is not properly monitored and evaluated by experts, the programme is bound to be failed. A total of n=60 respondents were asked on their level of understanding about capacity building (Programme management, AIDS vaccine initiative, M&E etc.) and 5% and 95% of the respondents say that their understanding level is good and fair respectively.

As far as government services are concerned respondents are contented with the following services, Needle and Syringe Exchange Program, Provision of ART and clinical test services. In the NGO sector respondents are happy with their services like Prevention,

Table 2.12 Percentage level of understanding about the various components of NACP III

Programmes	Very good	Good	Fair	Total
Prevention (T.I, STI Care, ICTC, Blood Safety, IEC, Condom promotion)	00%	81.7%	18.3%	100%
Care (Treatment of O.I, Provision of free DOT treatments, PEP, ART)	00%	28.3%	71.7%	100%
Collaboration (GIPA, Inter sectoral collaboration, Involvement of ministries, workplace intervention etc.)	00%	11.7%	88.3%	100%
Capacity building (Programme management, AIDS vaccine initiative, M&E etc.)	00%	5%	95%%	100%

Treatment and after care services. Most of all under RIAC, Drug detoxification program is well appreciated by the respondents.

Though NSEP is well appreciated, few complains about unnecessary harassment from the police as the police are taking undue advantage from people who carry used Syringe for exchange with fresh one by charging some money in the pretext of avoiding detention. It can be concluded that the respondents are happy with the services provided by the government and NGO's except for negligible number of respondents wanted government to provide Drugs for opportunistic Infections and subsidized the rates of basic necessities for people living with HIV and AIDS.

CHAPTER 3

Government and NGO's: Program Modalities and Implementation

The first initiative of the Government of India to take up the causes of HIV and AIDS was the setting up of National AIDS Control Program (NACP) in India in 1987. There has been four successive AIDS control programme. NACP I - 1992-97-99, NACP II -1999-2004-06-07, NACP III 2007-12, NACP IV-2012-17. Various strategies and action plans of the government have been discussed.

Some of the main objectives of the 12 NGO's as justified in chapter IV includes: Outreach work to different communities, HIV and AIDS awareness program, condom promotion, Needle and syringe exchange program, Home based care, referral services, DOT service at drop in centre, Coordination between various positive people, Advocacy, Helping children orphaned by HIV and AIDS, SHG formation for PLWHA, Women Empowerment, eradication of illiteracy by taking up various educational programmes, HIV and AIDS intervention programmes among C.S.W, IDU, MSM, developing a strategies for effective implementation of child rights especially of HIV and AIDS infected and affected etc. Some of the main strategies adopted by NGOs in HIV and AIDS mitigation interventions are peer-group approach, capacity building of the project personnel, condom promotion strategies, accessibility of IEC materials, STD diagnosis and treatment, outreach work strategies and intervention at the community levels.

MODALITIES OF GOVERNMENT PROGRAM PLANNING AND IMPLEMENTATION

The level of HIV prevalence varies across different states of India. The Government of India classifies the states of India into 3 categories based on the rate of HIV prevalence among clients of Ante Natal Attendees and high risk groups. The states of Maharashtra, Tamil Nadu, Manipur, Andhra Pradesh, Karnataka and Nagaland have been identified as high prevalence state because the HIV prevalence rates exceed 5 percent among high-risk groups and exceed 1 percent among antenatal women. The states of Gujarat, Goa and Pondicherry which share geographical borders with the high prevalence states report HIV prevalence exceeding 5 percent among high-risk groups but less than 1 percent among antenatal women and high prevalence state. Low prevalence states are those that HIV prevalence rate is less than 5 percent in high risk groups, and less than 1 percent among antenatal women. The Indian government initiative has not been discussed in detail here as it has already been discussed in chapter one. Only specific visions, aims and objectives are discussed in the present chapter.

The first initiative of the Government of India to take up the causes of HIV and AIDS was the setting up of National AIDS Control Program (NACP) in India in 1987. The Government of India through the Ministry of Health and Family Welfare set up National AIDS Control Organization (NACO) a nodal agency to take up the cause of HIV and AIDS in India.

NACP I

NACO launched the 1st NACP initially designed for five years, (1992-1997), but due to various difficulties in program planning and implementation, it was extended for another two years till 1999. The main focus of the 1st NACP was mass campaign on awareness. It was funded by World Bank and a strong WHO Global Program on AIDS (GPA) support. The ultimate objective of the project was to slow the spread of HIV to reduce future morbidity, mortality, and the impact of AIDS by initiating and establishing a comprehensive multi-sectoral program. The various components of the first phase were (a) Program management (b) Intersectoral collaboration (c) HIV and AIDS surveillance (d) Targeted interventions among high risk groups (e) Condom Programming (f) Sexually Transmitted Disease (STD) Program (g) Blood safety program (h) Information, education and communication (I.E.C) (i) Impact reduction

The outcome of NACP 1 has made awareness levels increased to about 70-80% in urban areas even though the level of awareness in rural areas remains low at about 30%; Modernization and strengthening of blood banks; introduction of licensing system of blood banks and gradual phasing out of professional blood donors; and availability of good quality condoms through social marketing has made a significant increase in its use.

NACP II

The 2nd NACP was also designed for five years, (1999-2004), and the program underwent a dramatic changes focusing on preventive intervention among targeted populations, institutional strengthening and inter sectoral collaboration. The 2nd NACP was also extended initially for two years till 2006 and was further again extended for one more year till 2007.

The policy and strategic shift was reflected in the two key objectives of NACP II. Reducing the spread of HIV infection in India, Increasing India's capacity to respond to HIV/AIDS on a long-term basis, Achieving condom use of not less than 90%among high risk categories like commercial sex workers, truck drivers etc., and Achieving awareness level of not less than 90 % among the youth and others in the reproductive age groups, Reducing blood borne diseases and transmission of HIV to less than 1% of total transmission. While the success of NACP II could not be undermine but there are complexities to be understood. There are Complexities of the epidemic and its exact dimensions which have to be understood especially in the Northern and North Eastern states of the country.

There is a frequent change of Project Directors (PDs) of State AIDS Control Societies (SACS) and other senior program managers at the state level which weakened the thrust and focus of interventions.

NACP III

The 3rd NACP was launched for another five years, (2007-2012), with the main focus of halting and reversing the HIV and AIDS epidemic in India by the year 2012. NACP III follows the strategy of unified three ones, one Agreed Action Framework, one National HIV and AIDS Coordinating Authority and one agreed National Monitoring and Evaluation System. The specific objective is to reduce new infection as estimated in the first year of the program by: Sixty per cent (60%) in high prevalence states so as to obtain the reversal of the epidemic; and Forty per cent (40%) in the vulnerable states so as to stabilize the epidemic.

The goal, objectives and strategies of NACP-III will be informed by the following guiding principles: The unifying credo of Three Ones, i.e., one Agreed Action Framework, one National HIV/AIDS Coordinating Authority and one agreed National M&E System. Equity as monitored by relevant indicators in both prevention and impact mitigation strategies i.e. percentage of people accessing services disaggregated by age and gender. Respect for the rights of the PLHA, as it contributes most positively to prevention and control efforts. NACP-III would evolve mechanisms to be put in place at all levels to address issues related to human rights and ethics. Particular focus would be on the fundamental rights of PLHA and their active involvement as important partners in prevention, care, support and treatment initiatives.

NACP IV

The fourth NACP is also design for five years 2012-2017 with an aim to accelerate the process of reversal and further strengthen the epidemic response in India through a cautious and well defined integration process over the next five years.

The goal is to Accelerate Reversal and Integrate Response and the objective to reduce new infections by 50% (2007 Baseline of

NACP III) and provide comprehensive care and support to all persons living with HIV/AIDS and treatment services for all those who require it.

The key strategies of NACP IV includes: Intensifying and consolidating prevention services, with a focus on HRGs and vulnerable population; Increasing access and promoting comprehensive care, support and treatment; Expanding IEC services for (a) general population and (b) high risk groups with a focus on behaviour change and demand generation; Building capacities at national, state, district and facility levels and strengthening Strategic Information Management Systems.

There are certain new initiatives under NACP-IV which includes: Differential strategies for districts based on data triangulation with due weightage to vulnerabilities; Scale up of programmes to target key vulnerabilities a. Scale up of Opioid Substitution Therapy (OST) for IDUs b. Scale up and strengthening of Migrant Interventions at Source, Transit & Destinations including roll out of Migrant Tracking System for effective outreach c. Establishment and scale up of interventions for Transgenders (TGs) by bringing in community participation and focused strategies to address their vulnerabilities d. Employer-Led Model for addressing vulnerabilities among migrant labour e. Female Condom Programme; Scale up of Multi-Drug Regimen for Prevention of Parent to Child Transmission (PPTCT) in keeping with international protocols; Social protection for marginalised populations through mainstreaming and earmarking budgets for HIV among concerned government departments; Establishment of Metro Blood Banks and Plasma Fractionation Centre; Launch of Third Line ART and scale up of first and second Line ART; Demand promotion strategies specially using mid-media, e.g., National Folk Media Campaign & Red Ribbon Express and buses [in convergence with the National Rural Health Mission (NRHM) now National Health Mission.

NON GOVERNMENTAL ORGANISATION MODALITIES OF PROGRAM PLANNING AND IMPLEMENTATION

Soon after the discovery of HIV and AIDS in India during the year 1986, NGOs and CBOs have been at the centre of response, providing a lead role in many states in building effective strategies for HIV and AIDS prevention care and impact mitigation. In districts and state that have turned around major epidemics, such as Manipur, Maharashtra, Tamilnadu, Nagaland, Karnataka and Andhra Pradesh, non-governmental and community-based responses have played a long-standing and crucial part in the success to HIV and AIDS mitigation.

NGOs and CBOs are recognized as being innovative and uniquely placed to access communities affected by HIV and AIDS directly, particularly the most marginalised and vulnerable. The importance of NGOs and CBOs in response to HIV and AIDS has been recognised but the capacities of these organisations and the quality of their programmes may be variable. In view of these, it is imminent that there is a clear need for the funding of NGOs and CBOs to be matched by support to develop and strengthen their organisational and technical capacity. This has been necessitated to maximise their potential and achieve sustainability and scale-up of effective responses to HIV prevention, AIDS care and impact mitigation.

Brief Profiles of NGO's

The term NGO includes many different types of organizations, from small local groups operating in a largely voluntary and informal basis, to large private development agencies with multimillion dollar budgets and thousands of paid professional staff. The present study was conducted among twelve NGO's which has been established at least or the last five years.

A brief descriptions of the NGO's is given below as discussed according to Sukai,T.B, 2010.

In order to minimize any biasness in selecting the sample, records and data's were first verified of the performance of the organisations for the last five years. The organizations have been in existent for the past 5 years or more. Some of the main objectives of the 12 NGO's have been elaborated below: Outreach work to different communities, HIV and AIDS awareness program, condom promotion, Needle and syringe exchange program, Home based care, referral

Table 3.1 Brief profiles of 12 NGO's

Jame of the organisation	Year of estd.	Main objectives	Challenges
ntegrated Women and 'hild Development (I.W)	1998	Outreach work for PLWHA to different communities, HIV/AIDS awareness, condom promotion etc.	Stigma and Discrimination
ndian AIDS Consortium I.E)	1998	NSEP, Home based care, condom promotion, referral services, DOT service at drop in centre	Mobilizing the community, t the program interesting and successful becomes the most challenging task
Ianipur Network of 'ositive People (I.W)	1997	Coordinating various positive people, awareness campaign on HIV/AIDS, Advocacy, Helping children orphaned by HIV/AIDS, SHG formation for PLWHA	Problems of law and order, s discrimination and condom promotion among the Muslir communities
Ieetei Leimarol Sinnai ang (I.W)	1989	Women Empowerment, eradication of illi teracy, HIV/AIDS intervention program mes among C.S.W	most of their clients are com sex worker and non brothel t is difficult to locate them anc freely about sex and sexualit general and HIV/AIDS in pa
ifeline Foundation (I.W)	1992	HIV/AIDS mitigation among HRG, Condom promotion, SHG formation, B.C.C and bringing about society with drugs free life.	Prevailing law and order pro resource constraint and non s actors having a stake.
ocial Action and Service Organisation (I.W)	1997	IDU intervention , intervention among MSM, Condom promotion, HIV/AIDS awareness program in the communities	Behaviour change, dealing w various distinct groups and p law and order situation

:ural Upliftment and :ervice Agency (I.E)	2001	Prevention of HIV/AIDS among IDU's and other HRG, SHG formation for income generation among the spouses and condom promotion, etc.	lack of sufficient funds to organise a community meeti seminars, workshops etc on t basis, which in turn tends to clients who can be changed
Vide angle social :evelopment (I.W)	1994	Strengthening harm reduction measures and minimizing the spread of HIV/AIDS, develop strategies for effective implementation of child rights especially of HIV/AIDS infected and affected	seeking support from the cor for tackling stigma and discrimination
'eople's Welfare Association (I.E)	2005	Making a better society free from social diseases like HIV/AIDS, T.B, etc	lack of voluntarism among tl people and especially among group
.EWS Community care entre (I.W)	1999	care and support services for HIV infected and affected people	lack of financial support, poo manpower, fear of stigma an discrimination, law and orde situation, low level of accept the remote areas
Aanipur Voluntary Health Association (I.E)	1998	one to one interaction, outreach services, OPD program, mobile health check up, advocacy program, network meeting, condom promotion, peer education training, focus group discussion.	to convince the client and the community for change
:RIPA Society (I.W)	1998	prevention of HIV among IDU's, their spouses, children, care and support services. According to the organization peer education and HIV/AIDS awareness in the community has been most successful among other strategies.	Irregularity of funds has beei major challenge

services, DOT service at drop in centre, Coordination between various positive people, Advocacy, Helping children orphaned by HIV and AIDS, SHG formation for PLWHA, Women Empowerment, eradication of illiteracy by taking up various educational programmes, HIV and AIDS intervention programmes among C.S.W, IDU, MSM, developing a strategies for effective implementation of child rights especially of HIV and AIDS infected and affected etc.

Strategies

Some of the main strategies adopted by NGOs in HIV and AIDS mitigation interventions are peer-group approach, capacity building of the project personnel, condom promotion strategies, accessibility of IEC materials, STD diagnosis and treatment, outreach work strategies and intervention at the community levels.

a) ***Peer-group approach*** – It is the involvement of peer groups in designing and implementing HIV and AIDS messages which make sure that the messages are more relevant to the community and acceptable by the high risk population. They often played a key role in gathering the beneficiaries for awareness camps and also building rapport among the staff and the beneficiaries. Peer educators in these projects are seen as facilitators and key influencers of the community.

b) ***Capacity building*** - Capacity building of the staff by regular training is one of the strategies implemented by most of the NGOs. Issues related to HIV and AIDS prevention, condom promotion, STD diagnosis, treatment and behavioral change communications, training programmes for the outreach staff included topics on approach and initiation of talk with the clients, and in understanding the clients' behaviour.

c) ***Condom promotion Activities*** – Condom promotion though not an established strategies in Manipur but are available in the chemist shops and various designated outlets. Besides free supply of condoms at the offices of the non-governmental organizations and the health centre's of the Government, it could be purchased in areas such as chemist shops, Pan shops, dhabas, hotels, transport offices, petrol pumps and the project offices.

d) ***Accessibility of IEC Materials*** - The IEC campaign which has been designed to create awareness and influence individual behaviour. Street plays, leela, cinema halls, pamphlets and posters were used as media in the interventions. IEC materials have been focusing on to communicate to the illiterate, low-income high- risk populations and most importantly the ignorant ones.

e) ***STD Treatment and Counseling*** – Almost all the NGO's gave importance for the diagnosis of STD through Syndromic recognition and the laboratory testing facilities. Counseling as such has been given utmost importance before testing and post testing.

f) ***Outreach Work Strategies*** – The outreach workers involve individuals both from high-risk population and general population. Outreach workers were given training in a specific manner with a set of specific education messages, devices and implemented by members of the community. The trained outreach workers know when, where and how to engage high-risk populations in the AIDS prevention campaigns. Outreach workers were trained to establish rapport building, and are also responsible for IEC materials distribution, dissemination of information about condom and STD diagnosis and treatment.

g) ***Community Level Interventions*** – Promotion of safe sex behaviour and eliminating stigma and discrimination about HIV and AIDS have been considered to be important indicators of behavioural change. As a communication strategy, materials have been printed in local languages and also with multilingual capacity. Some of the other main activities of the NGOs also include behavioral change through group educational session, providing information related to sex and sexuality, providing quality STD care, outreach services like home based care, helping community members to develop prevention strategies etc. Apart from these they also focus on building leadership at community level on different issues such as savings and credit, formation of women self help groups etc. However, with HIV infection and AIDS continuing to spread in India, a new and better approach for prevention and control is needed.

EVALUATION OF ONGOING PROGRAMME ACTIVITIES

In order to understand the ongoing program activities of the governmental and non-governmental organizations, two (2) functionaries each from twelve (12) NGO's and two (2) counselors from government ICTC centre were interviewed. Of the (12) organizations, 8 were from Imphal west and 4 were from Imphal east. Apart from the functionaries, one (1) Administrative head from each (12) organizations were also interviewed as they would be instrumental when critically analyzing the ongoing program activities.

There are varieties of programs being carried out by the non-governmental sectors in India. In the context of HIV and AIDS mention may be made of the ongoing programme activities in Manipur like Rapid Intervention and Care program (RIAC), Drug rehabilitation programs, Men who has Sex with Men program (MSM Program), Needles and Syringes Exchange Programs (NSEP) etc. The integrated RIAC program was launched on 7th November 1998. It is being implemented, at present, in collaboration with 45 NGOs covering all the 9 districts of Manipur. The objectives of the programme are:

(i) To minimize the spread of HIV infection among injecting drug users by making the IDUs accessible to clean needles, syringes and other injection works; education, counseling, skill development and referral network to drug treatment and other social support networks.

(ii) To minimize the spread of HIV infection from IDUs to female sex partners through condom promotion, education and counseling.

(iii) To monitor and evaluate the change in the behavioral pattern of the IDUs.

(iv) To help and support the people living with HIV and AIDS and to initiate community mobilization so that the families and community can take responsibility for care of people living with HIV and AIDS.

(v) To ensure effective linkage between community and hospital through formation of "Thoudang Marup" (community action groups) at the community level and Layengshangee Marup (hospital action groups) at the hospital or Community Health Centres and Primary Health Centres.

(vi) To provide home based care services for the needy patients and to produce a "Home Care handbook".

Making injecting safer for people who use drugs by providing sterile equipment is relatively easy and inexpensive and can significantly reduce levels of HIV transmission (UNAIDS Global Report 2010). The impetus for the creation and maintenance of Needle and Syringe Exchange Program (NSEP) emerged from the philosophy of harm reduction, an approach that assumes the probability of contracting or spreading HIV and AIDS is minimized by providing IDUs with clean needles at little or no cost. The establishment and maintenance of NSEP reduce the risk of spreading HIV and AIDS between IDUs as well as to their sexual partners.

On being enquired about supply of Needles and Syringes to 60 beneficiaries 83.7% said they receive Syringe regularly from NGO's where they are attached to. Heads of the twelve non-governmental organizations also replied in the affirmative that they promote NSEP as it is proved to be very effective in controlling HIV and AIDS.

Interestingly the secretary of All Manipur Anti Drugs Association (AMADA) said their organization was not of the opinion of promotion of NSEP at the beginning but later they uphold the idea after careful consideration and promote responsible use of it.

According to a study conducted by Sarin E., et al (2008), on working women who use drugs in Delhi, India. It was found that the biggest limitations in the design of drug treatment interventions in Delhi are that there is a lack of diverse treatment options for women users. Only indoor detoxification and rehabilitation facilities are available for women and even these has not been offering a quality of care which commensurate with the needs of the women. Lack of mental health care in drug treatment centres has been felt to be a huge gap in services. They conclude that NGOs like Sharan and Sahara are obliged to take up the entire continuum of care services which limits their ability to provide optimal care and services to women drug users. Lack of funds and lack of understanding among funding agencies about issues of women users are additional limitations in service provision.

The government ICTC centre where the counselors were interviewed is in the heart of the capital. The centre is located in the building of Regional Institute of Medical Sciences (RIMS) a premier medical institute being funded by the Ministry of Development of the North Eastern Region (DONER) Government of India.

Intervention programs for the sex workers both brothel based and non brothel based like spreading awareness on HIV and AIDS and condom use has a positive impact. In the present study Meeitei Leimarol Sinai Sang is the only organsation working with female sex workers. At present there are no brothel based sex workers in Manipur who are working in the industry. They function through different channels. Since there is no designated district at present like G.B Road in Delhi, Sonagachi in Kolkata and Kamathipura in Mumbai, female sex workers are unnecessarily harassed by the police commando's and other social organization, reported the head of the organizations. Apart from the harassment they got from these organizations they are in the very high risk groups as they cannot be intervened since they go underground. But to a great extent where ever organizations function they are able to change the behavior of the female sex workers. They educate them, provided them vocational training for income generating programmes and it can be said that it has greatly shaped their behavior to leads a normal life, according reports the head of the organizations. Similar success stories could be seen in a study conducted by Singh IP 1998 on STD-HIV intervention programme: the Sonagachi model. The study shows that sex workers awareness on HIV and AIDS increases from 30.7% at baseline in 1992 to 96.2% in 1995. The percentage of sex workers who always use condoms increased from 1.1% at baseline to 50.1% in 1995. The program has enhanced the self-respect and professional identity of the sex workers. As a result, sex workers are better equipped with the requisite knowledge and the courage to negotiate condom use with clients and to turn away men who refuse.

Manipur as is known by one and all in India is famous for its sporting talents and represented India internationally on many occasions. Sports have become a popular tool for HIV prevention, based on claims that it can foster life skills that are necessary to translate knowledge, attitudes and behavioral intentions into actual behavior. Many of the NGO's make use of the popularity of sports in the state of Manipur and the Manipuri's passion for it to spread awareness about it. Almost 90% of the total NGO's n=12 conducted their half yearly recreational activity by organizing a one day sports meet and going for outdoor picnic. According to heads of these organizations it has a positive impact to the service providers' i.e their staffs. It boosted their morale, increased their confidence level and productivity. It reduces their stress level and enables them to become friendlier with the clients.

Similar kind of impact of sports in HIV prevention programs could be seen in a study conducted by Delva W., et al 2010 on HIV prevention through sport: the case of the Mathare Youth Sport Association in Kenya. They conclude that though sports has a positive impact more rigorous evaluations of sport programmes for HIV prevention are needed.

Details of the ongoing programs were obtained from the respondents in the context of their organizations. Different program activities such as prevention education in educational institution, awareness programs in the communities, dissemination of I.E.C materials, provision counseling services and condom distribution activities were all discussed. Their opinion was also sought on the use of folk media such as Drama or Leela in their programs. Their responses are as discussed below.

The respondents were asked on whether their organizations gave HIV and AIDS prevention education in schools and colleges. Out of the total respondents, 76.9% of them state that their organizations have such programs. All of the functionaries reported of having programs such as counseling services, condom promotions and distributions and peer education. On the other hand only 38.5% reported the use of folk media in reaching out to the people. Probably their programs and strategies are so structured that there is little scope and may be timed for experimenting with creative methods using media such as drama or leela. Another 23.1% felt that peer education also to be one of the most successful among the many intervention programs. This can be substantiated by a study conducted by Van Rompay KK et al 2008, on development of an HIV peer education model for low literacy rural communities in India. The method employed was selection of six non-governmental organizations (NGO's) with good community rapport collaborated to build and pilot-test an HIV peer education model for rural communities. The program used participatory methods to train 20 NGO field staff (Outreach Workers), 102 women's self-help group (SHG) leaders, and 52 barbers to become peer educators. Cartoon-based educational materials were developed for low-literacy populations to convey simple, comprehensive messages on HIV transmission, prevention, support and care. In addition, street theatre cultural programs highlighted issues related to HIV and stigma in the community. The result shows that the program has reached an estimated over 30,000 villagers in the district through 2051 interactive HIV awareness programs and one-on-one communication. Outreach workers (OWs) and peer educators distributed approximately 62,000 educational materials and 69,000 condoms, and also referred approximately 2844 people for services including voluntary counselling and testing (VCT), care and support for HIV, and diagnosis and treatment of sexually-transmitted infections (STI). At least 118 individuals were newly diagnosed as persons living with HIV (PLHIV); 129 PLHIV were referred to the Government Hospital for Thoracic Medicine (in Tambaram) for extra medical support. Focus group discussions indicate that the program was well received in the communities and has led in the improvement of health awareness and also provided the peer educators with increased social status.

Further detail discussion with the respondents showed that 61.5% felt that HIV and AIDS awareness programmes in the communities seem to be the most effective of all prevention programmes.

Interestingly some of the respondents also report that peer education is a successful intervention strategy in their organization. This is quite obvious because at the community level outreach programs are for a larger audience. The success of community involvement and peer education could be substantiated by a study conducted by Maticka-Tyndale E and Barnett JP (2010). They critically review and synthesize the results and lessons learned from 24 evaluated peer-led programs with an HIV and AIDS risk reduction component that target youth in the communities where they live and are delivered in low- and middle-income countries. Interventions were identified through a comprehensive search of the peer reviewed AIDS-related literature as well as publication lists of major organizations in the UN family that address HIV and AIDS. The synthesis of the study results finds that these programs have demonstrated success in effecting positive change in knowledge and condom use and have demonstrated some success in changing community attitudes and norms.

There are different challenges faced by the functionaries while implementing HIV and AIDS prevention programmes discussed. Some of the most common challenges of the respondents were that they did not get full support of the communities due to stigma and discrimination attached to HIV and AIDS virus. According to some respondent discussion on the issue of sex and sexuality are taboo and not many people come forward to utilize their services. Another respondent mention that in his opinion the youth are also not very easy to reach out to. On the whole mobilizing the community to take part in awareness program is a big challenge. Not only this, a lot of creativity is needed in terms of use of appropriate media to make the program interesting and reachable to the masses.

Problems of law and order like the insurgency in North east and Manipur in particular which has been widely accepted as political and economic problem, frequent Bandhs and blockages called by various organizations fuelled by stigma and discrimination also create a great hindrance in HIV and AIDS intervention programmes that being carried out by various organizations. One of the organization in which one functionary were interviewed said that most of their clients are commercial sex workers and non brothel based; it is difficult to locate them and talk freely about sex and sexuality in general and HIV and AIDS in particular. The reason behind sex workers being underground has been due to unnecessary harassment by police commandoes and certain social organizations state head of one organization.

Among the 12 NGO's, 4 organizations received funding from foreign donors like Catholic Relief Services, Child Rights and You, Clinton Foundation and Childline. According to them funds from foreign donors has greater flexibility compared to funding from national and state government. The remaining 8 organization are being funded by NACO through the State AIDS Control Society.

Organizations which are not so well established, the administrative head had to shell out money from their own pockets to continue with their work when funds did not reach them on time. In response to a query on the success of alternative sources of fund raising conducted by these 12 organizations; selling of seasoned lottery tickets, organizing a Tambola game and charity shows are one of the most popular form. Charity shows though once a very popular one amongst the Manipuri's, it has not been successful during the present times where cheap video CD's are available in the market coming from Myanmar.

Irregularity of the funds being released by the state government hampers the continuity of the intervention programmes. Out of the total respondents 10 respondents did mention about lack of sufficient funds to organize community meetings and awareness program on timely basis. Most of the organization provides general health care to PLWHA, referral services; home based care and

STI TREATMENT AND MANAGEMENT

Another 12 respondents said their organizations provide HIV-TB co-infection management, 16 respondents said they provide Palliative (reducing the severity of disease symptom) care and 18 respondents said they provide Pediatric (infant and child care) aids treatment. The entire organizations have collaboration with other NGO's and care centre and they provide Nutritional support for people living with HIV and AIDS.

Table 3.2 various challenges in providing care and support services

Care and Support services	%age
general health care to PLWHA	11.5
palliative (reducing the severity of disease symptom) care, home based care	15.4
pediatric (infant and child care) aids treatment	3.8
nutritional support	7.7
any other	61.5
Total	100.0

In Table 3.2, it can be seen that various challenges faced by the respondents in providing care and support services to the people are different. Out of the total respondents 11.5% said that they provide general health care to PLWHA, 15.4% said they provide palliative care and 7.7% said they provide nutritional support.

There are different types of services provided by the nongovernmental organizations. Out of the total respondents 38.5% said they provide financial support, 7.7% said they provide financial support for ration or clothes, 61.5% provide vocational training to PLWHA. Most of the beneficiaries are not employed, so the organization gave training to the beneficiaries. Out of the total respondents 38.5% gave assistance in job Placement, 76.9% said they help the beneficiaries in self help group formation, 61.5% gave educational support for children affected or infected by HIV and AIDS and 92.3% of the respondents shared they facilitate formation of PLWHA network .

Table 3.3 shows that SHG for economic empowerment draws the maximum number of response and it is the most effective services provided by the functionaries according to them. Vocational training to PLWHA and facilitation of PLHA network draws huge response from the beneficiaries and the functionaries and attributed 23.1% and 26.9% each respectively in popularity.

Table 3.3 Services provided and its effectiveness

Services	%age
financial support for ration/clothes etc.	7.7
vocational training to PLWHA	23.1
self help group formation	30.8
educational support for children affected/infected by HIV and AIDS	7.7
facilitation of PLWHA network	26.9
any other	3.8
Total	100.0

Out of the total respondents 7.7% each said that they provide financial support for ration or clothes and educational support for children affected or infected with HIV and AIDS.

Different organizations provide different programme management services to the beneficiaries. The different types of programme management services provided by the organizations are

Information sharing through publication of journals, newsletter etc, Participation in planning process of MACS, capacity building programme for health care workers and community leaders, provide the services of resource persons, clinical research and social research.

Out of the total respondents 76.9% said, they have information sharing through publication of journals, news letter etc. Out of the total respondents 76.9% said they participate in the planning process of MACS programmes. Capacity building programs for health care workers and the community leaders are important components of program management and 92.3% of the respondents said they have the services.

Taking note of the importance of providing a resource person in program management services, 84.6% of the respondents said they have it. Since most of the organization does not have their own laboratory for conducting clinical research and taking into consideration of the fact that resources are constraint in the tiny state of Manipur, 92.3% of the total respondents said they don't conduct clinical research.

Since the present study focus on the social aspects of HIV and AIDS, social research plays an important role. Many of the organization directly or indirectly supported by Manipur state AIDS control society conducted many social researches for their own program components or for other purposes. Out of the total respondent 69.2% said they conduct their own research.

Since none of the organization provides clinical research, it cannot be seen in the table 4.4 of the many program management services being provided by the organization. The challenges and difficulties as described by the respondents of the clinical research ranges from funding problems to manpower inadequacy. Heads of the 12 organizations also cited problems of funds due to irregularity in releasing them on time by the state concerned authorities.

Table 3.4 Percentage of challenges and difficulties faced while providing services

Services	Percentage
Information sharing through publications of journals, newsletters etc	3.8
Participate in planning process of MACS	3.8
Capacity building programme for health care workers and community leaders	19.2
Provide the services of the resource persons	7.7
Social research	15.4
any other	50.0
Total	100.0

Interpretation of Table 3.4 above shows the varying percentage levels of challenges and difficulties faced by the respondents. Of the total respondents 19.2% said they faced difficulty in capacity building program of health care workers and community leaders. As told, capacity building for the community leaders involved in-depth information, education and communication and behavior change communication process so that they are fully empowered.

Out of the total respondents 15.4% said they have difficulties in carrying out their research work, due to non cooperation from the public, law and order situation of the state like constant strikes and blockades. Providing a regular well known resource persons for seminars, workshops etc involve a huge amount of money, so 7.7% of the total respondents say they have difficulty in it.

One of the most successful stories for HIV prevention programs in Thailand has been the distribution of condom and a wide spread message about it. Condom promotion and distribution model used by Thailand has been one of the world most successful stories. In the context of India and Manipur in particular, are they really successful in the prevention of HIV and AIDS? There are no social marketing programs of condom adopted by the said 12 organizations head being interviewed. There are various factors associated with it. Some of the main issues pointed out by these twelve heads includes: Social stigma attached to it, cost of the condom, societal values, ethics and norms etc. In one of the interview to administrative head of one organization pointed out that, if condom vending machine is installed then people won't go for it as it has social stigma attached to it. But he suggested that if Chocolate and eatables are also included in the vending machine then it will reduce stigma as anyone can go and get eatables and the condoms together.

The above cited problems in condom use and availability could be substantiated by a study conducted by Sarkar N.N., 2008 on barriers on condom use. He pointed out that several factors were associated with non-use of a condom during sexual intercourse. Their cost often posed a barrier to condom use for the poor, even in developed countries. In many communities, moral values, ethnic and religious factors also played a role. Among other social factors, gender inequality, lack of a dialogue among partners with regard to condom use, and the stigma attached to the condom could all lead to unprotected sexual intercourse. Personal factors such as aversion to the condom, consumption of alcohol or use of drugs prior to sexual intercourse, and anxiety and depression all were negatively associated with condom use.

IMPACT EVALUATION

Out the total 60 beneficiaries 23.3% feel that the services they received from the government are not adequate. Their discontentment ranges from supply of opportunistic drugs to provision of essential commodities as they could not procure their daily needs with their meagre income. However on the other side an overwhelming 76.7% feels that the government has done enough for them. Out of the total respondent 95% feels that the NGO they are attached with provided them with their necessary requirement and are contend with it.

Regarding condom availability, STI diagnosis and treatment facilities (Mobile Clinics), ICTC's centre, IEC Materials, Required number of hospital beds, officials from State AIDS control Society, ICMR, Notable person and 12 administrative heads of the organization gave their opinion upon it.

Officials from the state AIDS control Society were of the opinion that the state has sufficient services among the above listed services through their departments and various NGO's associated with them. However officials from the state ICMR Unit were of the opinion that the state requires more STI diagnosis and treatment facilities like the mobile clinics. Though the state had introduced Mobile clinics but it requires more number to cover the interior parts of the state. They also voiced their opinion about the requirement of more hospital beds apart from the existing one.

All of the 12 administrative heads agreed to the fact that condoms are available but interestingly one administrative head pointed out that the quality of the condoms being supplied through MSACS are of poor quality complains beneficiaries. One administrative heads pointed out that clients prefer to take condoms which have beautiful and attractive girls picture printed on it. All the 12 heads are of the opinion that the introduction of mobile clinics is a welcome note but the number should be increased. They said IEC materials should be printed in different dialects of Manipur so that the people have better understanding of the intricacies of HIV and AIDS. The two notable person interviewed supplement the opinions of the 12 administrative heads saying that the number of mobile clinics should be increased, ICTC centre should be set up in the remote far flung areas, IEC materials be printed in every dialects of Manipur and the number of Hospital beds, care centre should be increased.

Regarding the RIAC program being launched by MSACS the administrative heads of the 12 NGO's were affirmative that due to the introduction of RIAC program the rate of infection amongst the IDU has came down drastically. One administrative head pointed out the need to include more care and support services.

After careful evaluation of their programmes it has been highlighted that stigma and discrimination still prevails in the society though not openly. Opinions of the 12 administrative heads show that instances of stigma and discrimination towards PLWHA are few but it still prevails among the general population. Two administrative heads goes to the extent in giving example about stigmatized client. A woman widowed by PLHA husband - Now the in-laws don't like her as they think that she is going to claim the ancestral property. When she goes back to her parental house her brother's and sister don't like her because of her Sero status and also they think that she will have a claim in the family properties. Another administrative head said one woman (widow) came for admission in our center. Her in-laws don't want her anymore. It compels her to come forward to our center. One little girl who lost both her parents, she had a grandmother who use to take care of her. After the grandmother expired there were no willing relatives to take care of her. She (the child) was taken to our center and we supported her in any way we can. We administered ARV drugs and has been taking shelter in our care home.

The ground reality still prevails, one administrative head said to tackle the problem of stigma and discrimination there should be an in-depth research and studies upon it and showed to the policy makers about the ground reality. One administrative head was of the opinion that there should be moral policing and the culprit should be punished. Other heads of the remaining organization were of the opinion to raise in-depth awareness among the general population. Of all the ongoing program activities NSEP a part of the RIAC program has been the most successful and they hinted the need to introduce a specific program for women, children and the orphan in line with RIAC program. One of the administrative head said to tackle the problem of stigma and discrimination there should be a committee like crisis management group.

CHAPTER 4

Role of Social, Cultural and Faith-based Organization

Social and Cultural organizations plays an important role in the prevention and mitigation of HIV and AIDS. India being a culturally diverse country, having strong cultural ethics, norms and values, it can go a long way in the prevention of HIV and AIDS by making use of these cultural organizations.

Society is a type of social organization and that social organization refers to patterns of social interaction. Social organization is represented by the various parts of society in so far as they function with one another (Charon, 1986). Any group organized for a specific purpose becomes essential to social life or social order in the normal state of society; it becomes a part of the social organization. An organization is set up to achieve a certain purpose, to unite its members' activities and regulate them in the name of the given purpose. In its turn, organization's activities suggest its performing of definite functions.

The present study in Imphal shows that there are two main social organizations that play as a moral guardian to the society by promoting their objectives of a drug free society. As already discussed the first HIV reactive blood sample was found from a drug user. Manipur shares international border with Myanmar, from where all the drugs are coming to the border town of Moreh (Beyrer et al. 2000).

The two prominent organizations are:

(1) All Manipur Anti Drugs Association (AMADA) and

(2) Meira Paibi's

Both these organizations are known to have taken the initiatives of curbing the social menace of drug abuse in the state. They are instrumental in taking up the issue of social problem in the past also.

Contribution of All Manipur Anti Drugs Association (AMADA)

All Manipur Anti Drugs Association (AMADA) was established in the year 2005 with the main objective of helping people to lead their lives in a society completely free of drugs. During the time drug use was rampant among the youngsters. The period 2000 onward was one when drug abuse was very high amongst the youth (MSACS). AMADA a social organization started its services on HIV and AIDS by generating funds from the public. Initially their focus was only on curbing drug abuse and later they expanded their services to HIV and AIDS mitigation. The main programs organized by them towards HIV and AIDS prevention include seminars, forming health clubs and self help group. These has been regularly organized in the last few years

Two representatives of AMADA were interviewed for the purpose of the study. They reported the activities of their organization and its achievement.

There have been many success stories especially of AMADA in curbing drug use in the state. They associate themselves with other established NGO's for their technical and material support in their programs. In one incident a minor boy who was orphaned by their parents died because of HIV and AIDSs, AMADA opened an account for the boy and deposited Rs. 10,000 as fixed deposit. The money they said would help the boy in his quest for further education.

AMADA in their endeavour to self employment started making their own detergent powder, in which all the workers are widows who are HIV positive. These women would manufacture the detergent powder with the help and support of AMADA. They would then sell the product in the local market and the profit margin would go to them. The capital money used in the manufacturing of the detergent powder would be kept in the account of AMADA and reuse it for further production.

In an interview to the general secretary of AMADA on his view about the organization takes on Needle and Syringe Exchange Program (NSEP) one of the core components of Rapid Intervention and Care (RIAC) project of Manipur State AIDS Control Society. He said NSEP at the beginning was debated among the members of their society. Most of the members felt, it was rather promoting and encouraging drug use among the society. So, they were not promoting it at the beginning but later when they were educated about the positive impacts it had in different countries, they upheld the idea of responsible use of it.

According to Chawng., et al 1999

Mizoram is one of the north-eastern state of India with a population of 900000+ has a high number of drug user of which injecting drug users (IDU's) amount to approximately 5000+. Out of these, 70-80 percent indulges in unsafe injection practices till the mid-2000. As a result, there is a high rate of injection related abscesses and ulcers IRAU, 68 Percent incidence. Also, HIV transmission through sharing of injection equipments constitutes 45.6 percent of the total HIV+ cases. Since late 2000, a number of NGO's under the funding of Mizoram State Aids Control Society aggressively carried out NSEP among the IDU population. The present scenario has shown major positive changes. 70 Percent of contacted IDU's accepted and practiced safe injection practices; the incidence of IRAU has gone down to 4 Percent, and only 2-3 Percent of new HIV infections among the IDU population were reported during 2004.

In the history of AMADA, youngsters were hauled up for their drug abuse. They are then counseled for a behaviour change and sometimes when a repeater is being caught up, they inform their parents about their habits. In certain cases some of the highly addicted persons are referred to care homes being run for drug users.

The role of Meira Paibi's

The "Meira Paibi's" means women torch bearers and as is evident it is a women's organization.

Women's of this tiny state plays major role in diverse activities since early times. The contribution made by the women group in the state economy cannot be ignored. They are the main workforce of the state; the famous Khwairamband Bazar in the heart of the city is all taken care of by Women. From locally made handloom products, kitchen wares, handicraft products to different varieties of vegetables and rice can be found in this market. Rice cultivation is also mainly done by women groups of the state. What is perhaps most important is the tradition of collective action that Manipuri women have. Nupi Lan is a word that translates as "women's war". In 1939, women of this tiny north-eastern region organised an agitation against the British which came to be known as Nupi Lan. They held the British political agent confined for several hours, in spite of a bayonet charge by mounted police. The British could not conquer this region. During 1970s the women of Manipur rose again, this time to fight collectively, another battle - against alcoholism among the men. In what became famous as the "Night patrollers movement", woman in groups patrolled the streets after dark and either extorted a fine from men who had been found drinking or beat them up. They raided breweries and forced their closure. Earlier, in 1904 and 1925 too, women had resorted to collective action, against forced labour conscription and against arbitrary tax imposts respectively.

The Advent of the term Meira Paibis to bring about social change

The Literal Translation of the term MEIRA PAIBI's is women torch bearer. In Manipur the role of women in bringing about social change can be traced back to the pre British period when Manipur was under monarchical system. Women's movement emerged in a more organized manner with a creative ideology from the early part of the 20th century though movement could be traced back as early as 1904 which stir up due to discontentment, dissatisfaction and contradiction in the then society of Manipur. Women's movement in Manipur is norm oriented type and connected with reformations. The official origin of the term MEIRA PAIBI was from Kakching under Thoubal district in 1977. Meira Paibis are groups of like-minded women, philanthropic in nature with no formal sources of funding. Their work reflects that they are instrumental in bringing about social change, through social advocacy and social action.

Manipur was earlier known to be a male dominated society, where women had no say in the family. During the developmental stages, the Manipuri society, has witnessed different trends. Over the years, the womenfolk of the society became empowered. Within the umbrella of the Meira Paibis, the womenfolk stood together to fight against the likes of Alcoholism, Drug Abuses etc. etc, where the use of these was considered fashionable in the Manipuri society. Women in the family now have the courage to counter their husband if they came home drunk. They are present even in the smallest of locality in Manipur. After the success stories are learnt from certain localities, it mushroomed all over the state. The initial agenda of controlling Alcoholism graduated to controlling drug abuse, looking after the law and order in an informal way and for the development of the society at large. As one can see in newspaper and various journals, for a Manipuri society every new day comes with fresh agenda for survival negotiation. Coping of fear and management has been every day dinner table discussion for a household. The imposition of Arm Forces Special Power Act 1958, an Act which gives right to police and army personnel to shoot an individual on mere suspicion, truly it is a draconian act.

The popularity of Meira Paibis gained momentum after this Act has been imposed as police and Army personnel are constantly raiding ones house. During these course of action the Meira Paibis would stand together to protect those members who are innocent.

The role of Meira Paibis on controlling Drug abuse and Alcoholism

The Meira Paibi's of the state are stronger in their presence among the society comparing with the other likes of social organizations. Their presences are felt among the different sections of the society in every locality. Their main objectives and works include banning of all intoxicating drugs available in the market. In many occasion they hauled up alcohol and drug vendors, seize their products and burnt them down in front of the public and the media.

Mention can be made of one such organization called All Manipur Anti Drugs Association (AMADA) where their objectives complement with the Meira Paibis. This organization also works for the betterment of the society in which youngsters were hauled up for their drug abuse. They are then counseled for a behavior change and sometimes when a repeater is being caught up, they inform their parents about their habits. In certain cases some of the highly addicted persons are referred to care homes being run for drug users. The initiatives and steps taken up by Meira Paibi's (women torch bearer) are one and the same with AMADA except for the case that Meira Paibi's are located in every locality.

Given the ability of the Meira Paibi's,

They can be mobilize and partnered with the government agencies to mobilized the community and spread awareness about Drug abuse and alcoholism. Many a times large consignment of alcohol and drugs are seized from the vendors by the Meira Paibis and they burnt them down. They also treated the users and the vendors alike. When interacted with one general secretary of a particular Meira Paibi's, she said they started their organization 10 years before to help control the menace of drug use in the society. Apart from the many social problems they are involved in they tried solving different levels of family feud.

The traditional belief of promoting drug use by promoting Needle and Syringe Exchange Program still holds true for this organization. According to them, they organize seminars, meetings etc to educate the society in bringing about a change. Funding to both the social organization discussed above is a big problem. For the maintenance of the organization they go from door to door and seek people's donation. There are many examples of families whose son and wards were addicted to drugs that have changed their behavior after these social organizations interventions. Those are the types of families who are the largest contributors in cash or kind for the organizations.

Due to the intervention of these types of social organizations the rate of domestic violence and petty crimes has come down to a certain level. Encouraging, promoting and partnering with them would yield the desired results of prevention of drug use and promotion of peace in the society.

Meira Paibis in the fight for repealing AFSPA 1958

Mention can be made of one landmark achievement made by the Meira Paibis in the case of rape, torture and murder of Th Manorama by paramilitary soldiers in Imphal, capital of north-eastern Indian state of Manipur on Thursday, July 15, 2004. In a highly unusual protest, some 40 women stripped naked and staged an angry demonstration outside the Assam Rifles base to protest the death in custody of 32-year old Th Manorama. The state was in total chaos for more than a month. The outcome of the protest made by the Meira Paibis was that the Assam Rifles had to shift their base from Kangla the heart of Imphal city to outside the city.

The women of Manipur are highly politicized.

In another unique case of extra Judicial Killing on November 2, 2000, in Malom, a town in the Imphal Valley of Manipur, ten civilians were allegedly shot and killed by the Assam Rifles, one of the Indian Paramilitary forces operating in the state. A social activist Irom Sharmila Chanu also known as the "Iron Lady of Manipur" started her hunger strike for the removal of AFSPA 1958 since 2nd November 2000. There has been recognition from the international forum but 11 years has lapsed and the controversial Act has not been repealed. However due to her AFSPA has been partially removed in the Municipal area.

Meira Paibis in the fight against Human Rights Violation

The Meira Paibis are very much concerned with human rights abuses committed by the Indian government than they are with their rights as women. Consider these two contrasting incidents. In 1997, during a routine cordon and search operation, Indian Security Forces raped a woman, holding her husband at knifepoint outside the room while her seven-year-old son, bedridden with polio, witnessed the crime. For months, hundreds of thousands of Meira Paibis supported by human rights activists and organizations, protested on the streets of Imphal. Yet in 1999, a young woman was physically threatened with violent reprisal by community activists when she chose to be sexually involved with a trooper of the security forces. In this case, the public was widely sympathetic to the activists. Meira Paibis a women's association and one of the largest grassroots human rights movements in the region, comprising virtually the entire adult female population in every town and village. It is the watchdog of civil rights violations at the community level, initiating and engaging in campaigns against rights violations, such as arbitrary detention, cordon and search operations, and torture, committed by the security personnel of the federal government of India.

But in the true sense of word women do suffer very much from rights abuses because of their gender, and they are not accorded adequate protection. Increasingly, Indian security personnel assault women for their support of opposition groups as a means of demoralizing and insulting the community at large. The recent report by an organization, the Imphal-based Centre for Organization of Research and Education (CORE), suggest incidences of violence against women, including rape, are increasing at alarming rates.

Moreover, while the community still arbitrates most disputes according to local customary law, which is more gender equitable, parties who stand to benefit from them, are increasingly accessing Indian laws that are strongly patriarchal regarding issues such as inheritance. In customary law, rape is an offense punishable by death and ostracization of the rapist's family and judgment is passed by a local court of senior women who examine the victim. However, the way that modern Indian policies address rape is unnecessarily protracted and traumatizing for victims. Because of moral and social conditioning, local judges are often sympathetic to the "innocence" or "extenuating circumstances" of the perpetrator.

However, the Meira Paibis are little concerned with women's rights in and of themselves, and believe that they must "get general civil rights implemented first." This is perhaps the inevitable attitude of people in a situation of violent strife that has lasted for generations and where civil rights are routinely flouted. The tendency to dismiss women's rights is also likely due to the culture, which prides itself on the traditionally high status and prominent role of its women. Consequently, many women are reluctant to see themselves as objects of human rights violations particular to their gender.

There is a paradigm shift in the ideologies of the Meira Paibis from solving local and petty problems to the governance of Manipur. Different types of Meira Paibis manned different Ministries of the state Government in different directions. This Meira Paibis seems to be more engaged in banging Lamp Posts, tonsuring peoples' heads for 'heinous' crimes like polygamy, unauthorized elopement, drinking, solving family disputes, setting up small roadside huts for 'Round The Clock' security coverage, organizing Demonstrations as and when called for by other 'vested interest' groups etc. Indeed, Meira Paibis have contributed a lot to various social reforms, more productive developmental issues. If these Meira Paibis can organize huge demonstrations on human rights issues, certainly they can be expected to organize such rallies, demonstrations etc. for pressuring the Official State Government to create a more conducive atmosphere for investment and corporatisation of Manipur. Considering the work and achievement of the Meira Paibis, it is important to identify, engage and increase the capacity of community support structures to support young people on drug prevention behavior. The government should engage different law and policy instruments to support youth prevention initiatives on drug abuse. The government and various social organizations in Manipur should come together and foster networking among all the likes of social Organizations.

ROLE OF FAITH BASED ORGANIZATIONS

Win-Gallup International Religiosity and Atheism Index ranked India among the top 20 most religious country in the world during poll conducted in the year 2011-12. Likewise the impacts of modernization have led to the emergence of new religion, revivals and reforms among the contemporary Indian society. Within India, vast majority of its people are engage in ritual actions from early morning prayers motivated by religious beliefs systems. This has been the practice throughout generations across the spectrum of families and is continuously evolving. Religion, faith and beliefs system then has become the most important facets of Indian history and contemporary life. Organizations such as Hare Krishna Movement, The Brahma Kumaris, The Ananda Marga etc. among the many few have been instrumental in the spread of Indian spiritual beliefs and practices. Considering the religiousness of the Indian people the present study has been conducted in Imphal to ascertain the ground reality what faith based espouses and practices.

The present study will unravel what faith based organization across the globe espouses vis a vis the ground reality, successes and what more role it can play in the Indian context with special reference to Manipur state. For a clearer picture on what FBO really is, let's look at the definition...

Definition of FBOs

Faith Based Organizations (F.B.O's) are groups of individuals who have come together voluntarily around a stated spiritual or belief system that informs and guides their work together. FBOs range from small, grassroots organizations with simple structure and limited personnel to large, global institutions with highly sophisticated bureaucracies, wide networks, substantial financial resources, and significant human resources. (USAID- United States Agency for International Development)

Role of FBO's on HIV and AIDS mitigation

A policy to guide a Churches response to HIV and AIDS is complex, because it is not only an expression that guides proposed actions, but also represents a value statement that guides the lives and actions of its individual members. The policy therefore needs to be comprehensive in its coverage, distinctive in its perspective, and clear in its underlying values. It should benefit from earlier experiences in policy and practice, and incorporate current understandings of HIV and the context in which it exists. Aruldas V., et al 2008 made a review of policies and declarations on HIV and AIDS made between 2000 and 2007 by various churches and church bodies, in India and internationally. The text of each policy/ declaration was divided into categories, e.g. theological basis, rationale for response, church life, social response, healthcare response, youth concerns, etc. It was found that, though these policies are by FBOs of a single religion i.e. Christianity, there were distinct differences in terms of the scope of the policy, the emphasis given to different categories, relating to the socio-cultural and economic context, etc. Based on this analysis, they developed an initial framework for policy. The framework was discussed at several workshops for church leaders, and found to be useful for wider discussions, ensuring that different aspects were given opportunity for focus, and facilitate discussions. The review of policy and declaration by Aruldas., et al 2008 shows that Ideology, culture, social and other contextual differences do influence policies/ declarations, even when they are developed by groups (in this case churches) belonging to the same religion.

Sue Perry., 2002, made a review on the contributions of FBO s to the continuum of care of HIV and AIDS infected and affected people in 53 countries in Africa. Sue Perry reviews mapping studies conducted by the World Council of Churches over the last three years and other reports. The review indicates that three key elements are necessary for a balance response on HIV and AIDS prevention. Good leadership which creates commitment, Technical knowhow and accurate up to date information and Resources: both financial and human. Sue Perry gave an example, Light passes through the prism and this is refracted into a spectrum of colours. The incoming light represent responses and emerging light represents the different components of a consortium of care. The report said that health services are often concentrated in urban areas. FBOs operate in parallel to the government and fill the gap. International donor's funds government not usually FBO's, it is high time to acknowledge that the vast majority of FBO are non-partisan service providers. FBO's are in the forefront of care initiatives from the outset but when it comes to funding it has been sidelined for resources. Donors have given funding to corrupt government and ignored the FBO's.

Church and Indian government are partners in the fight against TB, HIV and diseases (Catholic Bishop Conference of India, July 8-9, 2008) with an objective of advocating cooperation, collaboration and networking to contain the virus effectively. This initiative of the government and FBO's could be a well cited example on commitment from the service provider.

FBOs can be influential in policy debates concerning the legal, ethical, and moral issues surrounding AIDS and human rights (Lazzarini 1998),

Religious taboos on sexual education have been harassing AIDS prevention throughout Latin America. The confrontation between the condom and abstinence or fidelity has snapped closed any possibility for negotiating joint strategies. It has polarized political stances that clash public opinion and counterattack official efforts for AIDS prevention (Farill., et al 1992).

> "... activists in HIV prevention programs need to purge themselves of their own prejudices and negative attitude towards religious institutions and engage them as partners in breaking the silence" (Iwere., et al 2000).

World Vision an International Christian NGO has been implementing innovative HIV prevention strategies in Asia among high-risk groups such as sex workers, truck drivers, migrant workers, fishermen, and injecting drug users. The group promotes a variety of prevention modalities, such as condom promotion and distribution, syndromic management of sexually transmitted infections, and behavior change. Some of its programs are regional and focused on cross-border populations, and some are active in non-USAID presence countries, such as Burma. World Vision also works with AIDS orphans and people living with HIV and AIDS in a variety of care and support programs.

Catholic Relief Services (CRS) a prominent FBO in India that has been spearheading the HIV and AIDS prevention programs since 1989, with an emphasis on care and support for people living with

HIV AND AIDS. CRS in partnership with many NGO's in India implement their prevention programs like MSM project, CSW project, IDU's Project etc.

The Islamic Medical Association of Uganda (IMAU) has taken the lead in educating Muslim religious leaders about HIV and AIDS in mobilizing their support in response to the HIV epidemic. Between 1992 and 1997, IMAU implemented the Family AIDS Education and Prevention through Imams (FAEPTI) project, which covered 11 of Uganda's 45 districts. In each district, five-day training workshops were organized for imams, their assistants, and volunteers known as Family AIDS Workers. Imams from 850 mosques in the selected 11 districts participated in the work-shops, and 6,800 community volunteers (one-half of whom were women) were trained. Workshop participants studied topics such as basic facts about HIV and AIDS, sexually transmitted infections, behavior change, safer sex, and principles of communication and counseling. In the first year, after objections from Islamic leaders, the topic of condoms was omitted from the workshop curriculum. After further dialogue, the Islamic leaders agreed that education about the responsible use of condoms, within Islamic teachings, was acceptable, and the topic of condoms was reinstated. A follow-up survey found significant increases in knowledge about HIV and AIDS in the project areas. Community members in the project areas also reported fewer sexual partners and increased condom use. (Kaleeba., et al 2000; Kagimu., et al 1998)

> "... The magnitude of AIDS epidemic problem in the ASEAN region is increasing significantly. The increase has to be controlled in time, otherwise, religious, social and economic development in the region will be hindered and disparities within and between ASEAN Member Countries will increase accordingly ... every individual has the right to have appropriate and right information on HIV and AIDS. Without having the information nobody will be able to prevent HIV infection, all Muslim Leaders in all ASEAN Member Countries have to be properly trained to use the IEC instruments and methods. The well-trained Muslim leaders will then play their important role in HIV and AIDS campaign in their respective community. The

Jakarta Declaration of Islamic Religious Leaders, December 1998.

Some of the main activities of FBO's across the globe and in India

Some of the main activities of FBO's includes: Counseling support groups for people living with HIV and AIDS and their families; Support groups for educating local communities about HIV and AIDS; Peer education programs which aims at prevention of HIV and sexually transmitted infections; Income-generation and vocational training programs for people living with HIV and AIDS and their dependents; Care and support programs for children orphaned by AIDS; Voluntary counseling and testing services; Alternative employment or income generation opportunities for girls and women who are vulnerable to or trapped in the sex trafficking trade; Hospice care; Drama or basic groups to raise awareness about HIV and AIDS, and to mitigate stigma; Other method of fighting against stigma associated with HIV infection within local communities

The present study

The present study on HIV and AIDS was conducted in Imphal and has taken a holistic view of the program, its approach and processes by focusing upon all the actors.

Given the situation in Manipur, the location of the proposed study, Imphal contributed the highest number of People Living with HIV and AIDS (PLWHA) among the nine district of Manipur (Manipur State Aids Control Society). Moreover there has not been any research on the social and cultural context or the modalities of program implementation and various roles of FBO's and stake holders in HIV and AIDS Mitigation

For combating the HIV and AIDS epidemic in Manipur, Manipur State AIDS Policy 1986 was launched taking into consideration the following objectives: a) to prevent the spread of HIV infection, both at the community at large and in the health care environment. b) To promote better understanding of HIV infection in order to protect and support those who are at risk of or vulnerable to infection. c) To ensure that treatment and support services both for those infected with HIV and for their family are easily available and accessible. d) To ensure that services are efficient, effective and evaluated. e) To mobilize and unify intersectoral action, community initiatives and NGO/CBO support network for better co-operation among the participating agencies against AIDS.

The north eastern states of India and Manipur in particular are beleaguered with conflicts in the form of General strikes, Protest demonstrations etc. State after state and country after country has a recent past or current involvement in some form of conflict or repression. Manipur being the border state to Myanmar which comes under the notorious golden triangle having a long history of Psychotropic substance use with opium and cannabis and pharmaceutical drugs use such as Buprenorphine or a cocktail with Antihistamine injections or sedative injection preparations like the Benzodiazepines coupled with sharing of contaminated syringes and needles, unsafe sexual practices under the influence of drugs is one of the most important factors making Intravenous Drug Users (IDU) as major sources of infection. Trapped in an insurgent-affected zone together with the poor health delivery systems, Manipur needs to perceive the epidemic as an impending disaster of colossal proportion and needs to partner with various Faith Based Organizations of the state in the prevention of HIV and AIDS.

The state of Manipur witnesses' external and internal conflicts every now and then and the consequences have been devastating, causing profound individual and collective trauma which has been compounded by poverty, and leaving behind huge numbers of widows and orphans and making them vulnerable to HIV and AIDS.

Conflict has an adverse devastating impact on the psycho-social, economic aspects of the individual. It increases sexual & physical violence, Refugees & internal displacement, rising poverty which in turn leads to sudden destitution & capital waste, Disintegration of social & physical infrastructures, increasing the rate of Famine & import dependence, disease spreads and increasing HIV prevalence, lack of development & annihilation, migration & brain drain, insecurity & loss of hopes

Sex, Faith, Condom and the world religious leaders take on it.

India as we know is of multi cultural and multi religious country where talking about sex is still a taboo. Studies conducted by Manipur state AIDS control society has shown that the trends of HIV and AIDS infection have now shifted from IDU'S to the general population through sex workers and others in Manipur.

So HIV and AIDS poses a new challenge to religion as sexuality is not openly sermon at the church Pulpit or the Temple or the Mosque in Manipur. Knowing well the main mode of transmission is sexual, HIV and AIDS intensify the tensions that are present around sexuality.

Most of the well known religions have had ambivalent attitudes toward sexuality. Religions have always been important forms of social control, especially in the area of sexuality. But many religions, especially in the past, also respected and even celebrated the powerful forces that come with sexuality, whether for reproduction or for eroticism. Some of the religious leaders said:

"To Tibetan physicians, AIDS is really something new, and the immediate cause is negative: sexual liberty... such a major illness or major negative event also has a karmic cause, no doubt. But I think AIDS also has a positive aspect. It has helped to promote some kind of self discipline." The Dalai Lama, 1994

"God loves you all, without distinction, without limit. He loves those of you who are elderly, who feel the burden of the years. He loves those of you who are sick, those who are suffering from AIDS. He loves the relatives and friends of the sick and those who care for them. He loves us all with an unconditional and everlasting love." Pope John Paul II, California September 1997

"For us, an encounter with people infected with HIV and AIDS should be a moment of grace – and opportunity for us to be Christ's compassionate presence to them as well as to experience His presence in them." Bishops' Conference of the Philippines, 1993

"Perhaps the AIDS crisis is God's way of challenging us to care for one another, to support the dying and to appreciate the gift of life. AIDS need not be merely a crisis: it could also be a God given opportunity for moral and spiritual growth, a time to review our assumption about sin and morality. The modern epidemic of AIDS calls for a pastoral response."-Bishops of Southern Africa June 1990

'In an ideal world we have hoped that everyone would be responsible about sex...that everyone would behave as we would have hoped they would do. Unfortunately, in the real world that is not the case and it is to fly in the face of ghastly fates to pretend otherwise. So we are going to have to teach people so-called safer sex, we are going to have to speak about condoms and seek to make it possible for people to have access to reproductive sexual health.' Archbishop Emeritus Desmond Tutu

As truly said by Desmond Tutu the ideal world and the real world are real wide apart. Particular questions to young boys and girls who are sexually active from 60 respondents having diverse backgrounds from the age group of 17 to 30 years were asked on whether they have had sexual experience before marriages, in the present study.

The present study was conducted across four prominent faith based organizations and covering 12 NGO's in and around Imphal east and west district that are directly or indirectly supported by Manipur State AIDS Control Society. All the organizations were in existent for more than five years and have the repute to reach their targets in HIV and AIDS mitigation. Five respondent/ beneficiaries were selected from each organization and the report showed that more than half of the respondents reported of having sexual experience before marriage. A little lower than half of the respondent's report of not having experience it and some didn't give a response.

Out of the 60 respondents among the beneficiaries from services provided by NGO's, 68.3% were male and 31.7% were female. More than 11% of the total respondents were in the age group of 21 showing the highest number and most sexually active age. The second highest groups were in the age group of 18 and 25 which forms a little above 6% of the respondents. Out of the 60 respondent,

57 responded on the question whether they are HIV positive or not. 10 respondents said they are HIV negative which forms 17.5% and the other 47 responded that they are HIV positive which forms 82.5%. The mean age of the respondent was 33.3, 24 as minimum age and 50 as the maximum age. Out of the 60 respondent 33 of the respondents were earning in various capacities. The mean income of these 33 respondents was Rs. 4207.52 with Rs. 1500 and Rs. 8000 as Minimum and Maximum salary/wages respectively.

Of the four faith based organizations their main objectives in the containment of HIV and AIDS were, Rehabilitation of the drug addicts and alcoholics who are vulnerable to HIV and AIDS, CSW, MSW, MSM targeted intervention projects, Relieving the emotional pain caused by HIV and AIDS, Orphan and vulnerable projects. The strategies adopted by the four FBO's on BCC were holistic counseling through the teachings of Christ. Personal views on condom of the leaders who were interviewed shows that though they don't practically promote the use of it openly but they are not against the responsible use of it for protection from various infections. In reply to a particular question on HIV prevention policy, where others faith organizations the leaders would like to see, they said people should own the responsibility and there should be regular meetings and networking of various FBO's. The greatest contribution of FBO's according to these leaders would have been the changes which are visible among clients, changes in the behavior and risk perception among the church leaders and the beneficiaries. Among the problems voiced in the HIV and AIDS prevention program by the leaders includes that, clients are attentive to the program due to their addiction to drugs, less cooperation from the government, frequent bandhs, general strikes due to law and order problem of the state. Financial constraints for few organizations were also a big problem in timely intervention. Of the four FBO's leaders from two FBO's said that they are adequately funded.

Out of the four FBO's two of them totally abhor the idea of condom promotion, they stick to the classical idea of total abstinence. The other two despite not totally detesting the idea spoke about having safer sex practices and to be patient until marriage. They do not openly distribute condoms but spoke about it directly or indirectly withholding the importance of it in the prevention of HIV and AIDS.

Some basic belief of many faith-based communities is that care for others is important and that the relationship between people is an expression of, and a pathway into, a relationship with God. In view of this, many faith-based communities believes in: Abstinence, if people are not married and sex within a faithful marriage only.

Leaders from the four Faith Based Organization's in Manipur shows that they have ambivalent attitudes towards sexuality, faith and condom promotion. Despite the fact that condom promotion and distribution is one of the most effective ways of HIV and AIDS prevention strategy followed by many countries and faith based organization across the globe, of course with modification to suit the particular faith teachings.

Myths and misconception

Faith-based organizations across the globe (and in the wider community) thought that talking about sex may: Result in increased promiscuity; Seem to condone sex outside marriage and encourage immature and young people to have sex earlier

It is also believed that promoting condom use results in people practicing 'unacceptable's sexual behavior rather than abstinence. However, research has shown that educating young people about sex, HIV and AIDS and health in general does not result in increased sexual activity, but leads to a decrease in adolescent sex, unwanted pregnancies and STIs.

Contribution of FBO's in behavior change and the need for partnership

Data collected from 60 respondent's shows that more than half relapsed again due to lack of activity, idleness, frustration, depression, lack of self control and the will power after going through drug detoxification program. Whereas in the case of faith based counseling approached, the cases of relapse are negligible. So, it can be said that behavior change through Faith Based counseling has proved to be more successful than the other traditional methods. To maintain a stable or declining national HIV sero-prevalence rates studies has shown the importance of commitment from the leadership and open discussion about HIV and AIDS and partnership of FBO's and religious leaders. India being a highly religious country and in Manipur where FBO's constitute a major part of the nongovernmental sector, the government can engage them in the prevention of HIV and AIDS taking in examples of countries where FBO's played a positive role in stabilizing the HIV sero-prevalence rates. FBO's has the potential and the needed resources to reach out to the people. Religious leaders often interact with the community masses in the church, Satsang, Temple or the Masjid in Manipur. The government can make use of the fact that a leader of these groups has a mass appeal and they would be instrumental in HIV and AIDS prevention programmes in the state.

Study conducted within the aforesaid four FBO's whose approach to behavior change is through holistic counseling shows that Behavior Changes through these counseling has minimal cases of relapse than detoxification/ substitution model where the cases of relapse cases sky rocketed.

Case study example on the positive impact of holistic counseling in Manipur, *Mr. Tomba* age 37 years was a drug addict for almost 15 years. He was thrown out of his house for his addictive habit. There was no one to take care of him. He has no money, no roof over his head; he was lying and sleeping on the roadside pavement until he was discovered by one church pastor of the area. The time he was discovered he was in no position to stand or eat anything as his whole body was covered with abscess cases due to various infections. The pastor then enrolled him in one NGO who are working on drug rehabilitation program and HIV and AIDS prevention. As told he has no will to live in the beginning when his HIV serostatus was discovered. The pastor continues his visits and patiently counsels him. When the pastor told him that every person in the world is born with a purpose and nobody will continue hating him if he changed his past behavior. Mr. Tomba then begins to have faith in God that he cares for every one irrespective of what they are.*

He is a changed man now and runs an FBO successfully with the help of donations from the church and the people who are reformed after his program intervention. *Mr. Tomba name changed to protect identity

"BCC aims to foster positive behavior; promote and sustain individual, community, and societal behavior change; and maintain appropriate behavior" (FHI). As well said HIV and AIDS is a pandemic which forces societies to confront cultural values and practices that can contribute to the risk of HIV infection, effective BCC is vital to setting the tone for compassionate and responsible interventions.

It can also produce insight into the broader socioeconomic impact of the epidemic and mobilize the political, social, and economic responses needed to mount an effective program to address the epidemic. Example of a faith based organization on how they contribute to behavior change in Manipur with special reference to Christianity:

- Children advocacy programme: All the established churches in Manipur have a Sunday school classes. FBO's advocates the importance of HIV and AIDS awareness among the children's during these classes and taught them on how healthy behavior will give them the thrust in life and save them from various diseases.
- Youth Support Structures at Community level: FBO's made use of the church youth services and promotes the ideology of safer sex practices as they are in the most sexually active age group.
- Parents Capacity Building: Various FBO's in the Imphal area partnered with the churches, counseled the leaders and made them understand the importance of advocating the right attitude to life and to be united in the fight against various social problems such as social discrimination and exclusion of the less privileged sections of the society, HIV and AIDS etc.
- Community Capacity Building (leaders): Faith based organization tries to collaborate with local clubs and various stake holders and conducted various community sensitization program

- Peer Approaches: This is also one of the most successful strategies for behavior change. FBO's conducted focus group discussion among the peer groups, helped them in forming SHG's and conducted holistic counseling following Christ teaching for behavior change. Communication interventions that promote engagement and dialogue particularly among the peers – have been the key for changes in behavior. Singhall, A and Rogers, E M (2003)

Faith-based organizations are effective tools in responding to HIV and AIDS. FBO's involvement contribution in Uganda "... changes in age of sexual debut, casual and commercial sex trends, partner reduction, and condom use all appear to have played key roles in the continuing declines" (Hogle 2002). FBO's constitute perhaps the largest institutions in the world with the greatest built-in infrastructures of leadership and fellowships. Religion can build upon its moral and value-based leadership as they garnered trust over generations, and channels of communication and organization, in order to have a tremendous influence over cultural norms that guide individual and community behavior. Taking into consideration on how FBO would have tremendous impact in the control of HIV and AIDS the government of Manipur can seek partnership with them to contain the spread of HIV and AIDS. Communication approaches based on the assumption that individuals make rational choices about their behavior cannot effectively address the complex social character of HIV and AIDS. If faith-based groups wish to move towards open discussion about sex it is important to acknowledge that: there is more sexual activity happening in communities than they might readily accept, much of this sex is unsafe (as well as unlawful and unacceptable in churches' eyes) and not all 'lawful' unions are safe.

It is important to identify, engage and increase the capacity of community support structures to support young people on HIV and AIDS prevention behavior. The government should engage different law and policy instruments to support youth HIV and AIDS prevention initiatives. The government and various faith based organization in Manipur should come together and foster networking among all Faith Based Organizations

Looking into the success and achievement of FBO's in the state of Manipur the state government through its various agencies can Identify certain FBO's who are really doing well in their own part despite the size of the organization and fund their project so that the HIV sero-prevalence rate is reversed.

For example, the US Government through USAID has been funding FBOs such as World Vision, the Salvation Army, and Catholic Relief Services, awarding contracts on the basis of technical competence and experience in carrying out similar projects. In USAID's view, FBOs are a type of private voluntary organization that USAID funds because they bring experience, their own funds, and a record of achievement to international health and other sectors of development.

Research has also shown that however great efforts have been taken up by the state government to partner with FBO's the latter doesn't agree with the terms and conditions of the state government especially on condom promotion and certain other issues.

Some of the major issues would probably be to hire extra staff to carry out new or additional social services. Yet with the irregularities and uncertainties of government funding, FBOs would have to do just as much laying off of staff and new hiring, condom promotion etc. Some FBOs have used this as a reason not to become involved in the first place.

Whatever it might be, taking advantage of the success rate of the FBO the government should be flexible to faith based organization. Religious organizations ought to be given support to implement their "comparative advantage," i.e., promoting what they call fidelity and abstinence. And that is precisely what most of these organizations want to emphasize. Forcing FBOs to work in condom promotion risks alienating them from AIDS prevention efforts, and thereby losing the great potential they bring to such efforts. Community-based programmes, including income-generating projects, improved life skills, such as training youths in home based care and support to orphans, should be strengthened.

CHAPTER 5

Political Commitment: Realities and Issues

Needless to say, for an effective response to the HIV and AIDS pandemic, it requires the support and involvement of leaders from all levels and sections of the society. It is important and necessary to create a supportive environment for HIV and AIDS programs to be effective. To create such an environment it requires the involvement and mobilization of a broad political consensus that such programs are necessary for the well-being of the society. Mere formulation of appropriate policies and the allocation of resources will not yield the desired result. Political support can be broadly defined to include the involvement of senior government leaders and civil servants. Political commitment state indirectly support of a broad range of civil and community leaders, at all levels of the society. This includes the public sector, the private sector, nongovernmental organization (NGO), religious leaders, and other influential citizens at national and local levels. Leaders are the role models of a society and their personal actions and behavior send strong signals about what is important.

Political commitment is a concept which is difficult to measure by a data which are collected routinely. Commitment is also multidimensional and therefore, cannot be measured through a single quantitative indicator. It might be possible to measure commitment directly if leaders were willing to submit to regular interviews about their level of understanding and support for HIV and AIDS programs. Even in this case, there can be doubts about the sincerity of their answers. In this study political commitment has been measured indirectly by examining the statements, policies, and actions of leaders, what they have talked about HIV and AIDS or by what they actually do in varying degrees. It was seen that leaders who spoke out publicly about the importance of HIV and AIDS are expressing a commitment to the issue and creating a climate that encourages solutions. It was also learnt that for an effective response, it is also necessary for leaders to establish enabling policies, propose and support programs, provide funding, appoint good people to key positions, demand accountability, and participate in regular program reviews and evaluations. To actually find out realities and issues of political commitment, it has been discussed in various different topic heads

In order to find out commitment of the political leaders, a set of different questions were asked. Question ranges from policy making to program implementation and their involvement at the grassroots level taking into account not only the levels and degree of knowledge but also at the roots of the potential ignorance.

HIV/IDS POLICY AND ITS DIRECTION

As the first few cases of HIV infection of the country were reported in 1996, the Manipur State Government also took serious note of the problem and initiated a series of important measures to tackle the epidemic. The first HIV and AIDS case in Manipur was detected in1989 from a blood samples collected among IDU's in 1988. With the formation of the high-powered National AIDS Committee in 1986, Government of India launched National AIDS Control Program in 1987. In the year 1989 with the support of WHO, many other activities were initiated which were mainly focused on the reinforcement of program management capacities as well as targeted IEC and Surveillance activities. Actual preventive activities like implementation of IDU focused prevention intervention, education and awareness program, blood safety measures, control of hospital infection; condom promotion to prevent HIV and AIDS, strengthening of clinical services for both STD and HIV and AIDS gained momentum only in 1992.

Commitment of the state for development with other key societal actors being willing participant (i.e. political settlement is committed to development) for HIV and AIDS mitigation. Capacity of the state to implement policies effectively and this capacity being determined by other constituent capacities like the Institutional, technical and political. State AIDS Cells were created in Manipur for effective implementation and management of National AIDS Control Program. In 1996 the Manipur State AIDS Cell (MSACS) became Manipur State AIDS Control Society registered under Societies Act and it became an autonomous body with the objectives of reducing the spread of HIV infection in the state and to increase the state capacity to deal with the epidemic in the long term. Most of the programmes launched in the field of HIV and AIDS are with the help of MSACS, NACO and NGOs. The external agencies gave more emphasis on Prevention with minimum attention on treatment, care and support.

For combating the menace of HIV and AIDS in Manipur, Manipur State AIDS Policy 1996 was launched with following objectives:

a) to prevent the spread of HIV infection, both at the community at large and in the health care environment.

b) To promote better understanding of HIV infection in order to protect and support those who are at risk of or vulnerable to infection.

c) To ensure that treatment and support services both for those infected with HIV and for their family are easily available and accessible.

d) To ensure that services are efficient, effective and evaluated.

e) To mobilize and unify inter-sectoral action, community initiatives and NGO/CBO support network for better co-operation among the participating agencies against AIDS.

The Manipur state AIDS Policy has policies on various dimensions such as

a) Policies on Information Education and Communication,

b) Policy on school AIDS education.

c) Policy on Blood Safety,

d) Policy On Medical Care,

e) Policy on Std And Reproductive Health,

f) Policy On Drug Abuse Treatment Service,

g) Policy On Hospital Infection Control,

h) Policy On Intervention Measures,

i) Policy On Employment,

j) Policy On Antibody Testing,

k) Policy on Confidentiality,

l) Policy In The Prisons/Jails,

m) Policy On Social Service Research,

n) Policy On Non Discrimination Provision, o) Policy On Training and

p) Policy On Appropriate Legal Framework.

In order to facilitate speedy and proper implementation of the AIDS control programme, the State Government created appropriate bodies such as State AIDS Committee (SAC) with State Empowered Committee (SEC), and State Level AIDS Co-ordination Committee (SCC). It also created grass root infrastructure by creating District AIDS Committee (DAC).

Manipur stands out to be a state which has a specific policy on HIV and AIDS since 1996, and the direction it has given to AIDS programming in the state could well be analyzed out of the responses given by the politicians and the beneficiaries. Of the many program activities being carried out by MSACS, Targeted Intervention program for Injectible drug users called Rapid

Intervention and Care project has been one of the most successful. The number of HIV positive who are Injectible drug user has come down to around 16% in the state (MSACS). Maximum number of the respondent said that the number of IDU has drastically come down since the inception of Manipur state AIDS policy.

Certain aspects of the responses showed that though the policy has a great impact especially for the IDU's but there are loopholes as these response shows "*there are many programs, but they said it didn't reach the specific targets at the hills*". Notwithstanding the positive impact it gave in the control of HIV and AIDS the policy needs a serious relook. The policy has given a new direction and new strategy in the control of HIV and AIDS. "*It has given us a new impetus in the fight against HIV and AIDS*".

Positive development in the new revised Manipur State AIDS policy 1996

- Manipur state government will now allow utilization of MLA Local area Development Program (MLA LADP) fund.
- Introduction of District AIDS Prevention Control Unit (DAPCU)
- Inclusion of one male and female PLWHA in MSACS Committees
- Policy for involvement of CBO, FBO, Social Organization only for IEC Programs
- Compulsory training for student for two days to be eligible to appear for Xth and XIIth exam and teacher for three days to enter into state service.
- Provision of free travel for PLWHA
- Provision of Opportunistic Infection drugs
- Monitoring and Evaluation once in every year

INFRASTRUCTURAL, INSTITUTIONAL, MANPOWER AND SERVICE AVAILABILITY

It is a fact that very few hospitals in India are equipped to treat HIV and AIDS patients, and even in these hospitals HIV positive patients are often held at arm's length. The majority of "AIDS wards" in Indian hospitals consist of 1 to 2 beds relegated to a dingy and often filthy corner of the hospital, but the situation is now slowly improving.

On 15th March 2005 His Excellency Dr. Shivinder Singh Sidhu the then governor of Manipur in his speech at Manipur legislative assembly (proceedings Vol. 72 Appendix A 18) said the following points showing the state commitment in health care set up:-

> "My government is aware that HIV/AIDS is a major health concern in the state. Accordingly the State Aids Control Society is gearing up to face this new challenge. The Bill & Melinda Gates foundation has recently launched project ORCHID covering Manipur and Nagaland to support the efforts of the state government".

> "My government is now giving special emphasis to strengthening of medical infrastructure by sourcing additional funds from (Department for the development of the north eastern region (DoNER) and North eastern Council) NEC. Government of India has sanctioned Rs. 149.92 lakhs for up gradation of emergency & Accident services of Jawaharla Nehru Hospital. Construction of Trauma Centre is at an advance stage. Construction of 100 bedded hospital at Thoubal costing about Rs. 24.00 crores funded by the Urban Development Ministry is being started".

DoNER has retained schemes for Rs. 826.70 lakhs for strengthening of Health equipments of the district hospitals and 5 CHCs in the State.

The NEC has approved schemes worth Rs. 13.55 crores for strengthening of J.N Hospital, Churachandpur District Hospital and for construction of a nursing school with hostel, during 2004-2005. The state obtained ACA of Rs. 2.00 crores for improvement of the district hospitals in the hills and the scheme is nearing completion.

Construction of health centre at Moreh under BADP has been completed. The construction of a 50 bedded mental hospital at chingmeirong has started during January 2005.

In reply to a particular question on the availability of medical infrastructure like (number of hospital Beds, availability of trained medical professionals, requisite no. of ICTC, ART Centre, sufficient supply of screened blood, etc) shows that the state needs to allocate more funds for medical infrastructural improvement.

Further analysis of the responses shows that there should be more medical centre's to cater to the needs of the people who are living far flung from the city. Shortage of manpower like trained medical professionals to especially cater to the needs of people living with HIV and AIDS was also highlighted. One of the response says that "*more service personnel be included like social workers in the hospitals, up gradation of the infrastructure, etc*".

MANIFESTO ANALYSIS OF POLITICAL OUTFITS OF THE STATE

Manifesto, it is a public declaration of the intentions and promises made by a political party released well in advance by the party to seek the support of the voters. All the political parties of the state do have mention about people living with HIV and AIDS. With the exception of few parties of the state, politician do mention about protecting the rights of PLWHA. Political parties, be it the left wing or the right wing, socialist or democratic of the state talked about protecting the rights of PLWHA. Congress party goes to the extent of saying that they have it in their manifestoes of halting and reversing the spread of HIV and AIDS. A socialist party of the state response indicates that manifestoes should not only be in paper and goes to the waste bin the next day. It should rather be implemented as promised. The response says that "*Manifesto shouldn't only be in paper it should be properly implemented as is promised*".

MANIPUR LEGISLATOR'S FORUM ON HIV AND AIDS

UN General Assembly Special Session on HIV and AIDS (UNGASS) meeting in 2001 was a significant milestone in the political response to HIV and AIDS in India. Understanding the gravity and seriousness of the HIV and AIDS pandemic a parliamentary forum on HIV and AIDS was formed under the leadership of Mr. Oscar Fernandes on March 2000 at the national level as a convener. With the support of UNAIDS and in line with the Parliamentary Forum on HIV and AIDS, the Manipur State legislative Forum on AIDS was formed under the leadership of (L) Dr. S. Budhichandra Singh, the then Speaker of Manipur Legislative Assembly and Dr. I. Ibohalbi Singh, MLA as the Chairman and Secretary of the Forum respectively on 30th June 2007 with the following broad objectives: Reducing the gravity of stigma and discrimination, Awareness generation to the MLA's and Local leaders by holding seminars, workshops etc for the community. Containment and raising awareness on HIV and AIDS among the legislative members and state free of health problems.

Since the formation of the forum there has been no looking back and started their work by visiting the AIDS patients in community care centre's of "Best Practice Sites" in Imphal & Churachandpur on 22nd & 24th November, 2007.

Out of the many initiatives undertaken by the forum mention can be made of the followings: The MLFA joined the observance of World AIDS Day under the theme "Stop AIDS-Keep the Promise-Leadership" on 1st December 2007 with a mass rally on the streets of Imphal.

The MLFA in collaboration with the Rural Development & Panchayati Raj Department of Manipur organized a One Day Convention on HIV and AIDS for the Panchayati Raj Institutions (PRIs) on 29th December, 2007 at Imphal. The Chief Minister of Manipur, Shri Okram Ibobi Singh was the Chief Guest, (L) Dr. S. Budhichandra Singh, Speaker was the President and Md.Allaudin Khan, Minister for RD & PR was the Guest of Honour.

As a follow-up action, the Manipur State Panchayat Forum on HIV and AIDS was formed on the 16th Jan, 2008 with 14 members with the President of Manipur State Panchayat Parishad as its Chairman.

The state government under the aegis of Manipur State Legislative Forum on HIV and AIDS (MLFA) conducted a series of political conventions which involved members of the elected representatives of the state since January 2008.

The MLFA organize a series of political conventions during January, February and March 2008 at Konthoujam, Wangoi, Sekmai, Thanmeiband, Yaiskul, Mao, Oinam, Langthabal, Lilong and Sagolband to spread awareness to the people and educate the public leaders about the issue.

Shri TN Haokip, Minister of PHED, DIPR and Tourism, Manipur on behalf of the Manipur State Legislatures Forum on HIV and AIDS declared that the Antyodaya Anna Yojana popularly known as AAY will be made available to all people living with HIV and AIDS (PLHIV) in Churachandpur district at Saikot village in Churachandpur district on 9th August 2010 (Source: The Sangai Express). The Minister made this statement on the occasion; Manipur Legislators' Forum on HIV and AIDS (MLFA) constituency level convention on HIV and AIDS at Saikot in Churachandpur. A series of 60 such conventions will also be held in the near future in the remaining 59 assembly constituencies of the state.

Manipur legislative forum on HIV and AIDS plays an important role in spreading awareness by utilizing the forum to raise the issue in a bigger forum. The forum seeks the attention of the 60 members by conducting conferences, workshops, etc. among the legislative members. In a bid to hold 60 political conventions during their term, the forum already conducted a series of political conventions as an initiative to involve the people. The forum initiatives includes involvement of village chiefs, Panchayat leaders, religious leaders, local clubs and various stake holders in the fight against HIV and AIDS.

Involvement of politician's and its ministries in

a) Media

b) Opinion on the manner of surveillance and reporting on HIV/AIDS in the state

A total of eight politicians were interviewed representing different political parties of the state.

In order to find out the realities and issues concerning the state political outfit's commitment on HIV and AIDS mitigation, a self introduced semi structured interview guide was used. Interview guide

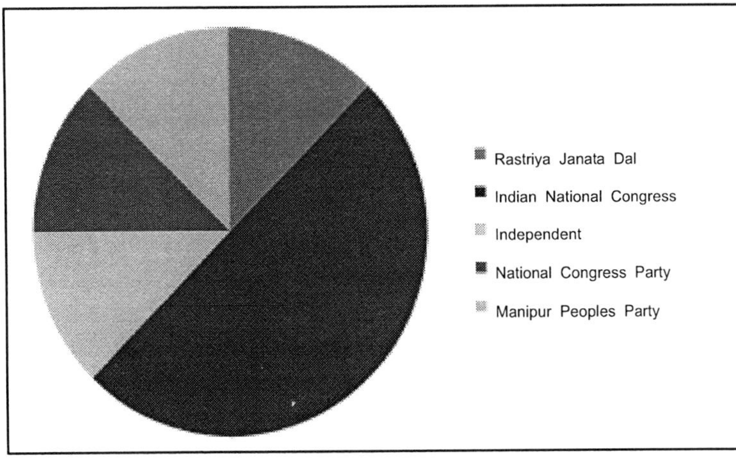

Fig 5.1 Pie chart representing different political parties

is a step by step guideline for the interviewer so that he does not miss out any important matter. Upon discussing a particular question, topics were elaborately discussed when required.

From the above pie chart, one can see different political parties. Leaders from different political parties were chosen to avoid any biases in their response, as leaders from only one political party would give the same lines of response.

The responses and viewpoint of the political leaders has been elaborately discussed to draw inferences and conclusions. Circumstantial evidence has also been taken into consideration and not only on the basis of direct observation but results which came out of conversation. Every issues and concerns which were discussed have been subdivided into topic heads constituting a topic of discourse.

Political parties and their leaders of the state consider HIV and AIDS as a political issue. It was noted that during the interview with the leaders there was a spectrum of opinion. Some of the responses went to the extent that "*it is not only political; rather it is also a social issue*". HIV and AIDS have engulfed the state of affairs as it affects all walks of life. One of the responses was that "*yes AIDS is a political issue as politics involves human issues so HIV is directly or indirectly related to HIV and AIDS"*. The formation of Manipur State Legislative forum on HIV and AIDS also shows that politicians of the state consider HIV and AIDS as a political issue.

Politicians are involved in various capacities in the legislative forum on HIV and AIDS. Their involvement is reflected through their work that has been done. There are members who have been invited as a chief guest in their constituency during a sports meet and spoke about HIV/AIDS awareness. Congress chief of the state hinted the scholar about the party and his individual involvement in many forums. He said that Congress party itself holds many awareness programs during the years gone by. Some of their activities include selecting and targeting some constituencies for raising awareness about the issue.

None of the politicians have any problem in their affiliation to a particular party on their stand with respect to social issues such as HIV and AIDS. One of the respondent cited he being an independent member doesn't affect his stand and spoke about the issue on various occasion. One of the responses was "*Not at all as it is a common issue for the ruling and the opposition party alike, we don't have any problem*". The responses show that politicians of the state consider HIV and AIDS not only medical or social but political as well.

INVOLVEMENT OF POLITICIAN'S AND ITS MINISTRIES

The Indian government's strategy for dealing with the pandemic emphasizes a comprehensive and decentralized approach. The pandemic does not only differ from one state to another and there may be dramatic differences from one district or village to another. The Indian government faces two main challenges which is integrating the response to HIV and AIDS with the rest of India's expanding public health goals and raising the budget for HIV and AIDS to a level which commensurate with the problem.

The government involved ministries other than Health and Family welfare like education, sports, transport and communication, etc so that the spread of HIV and AIDS is contained. For the best implementation of AIDS control policy in the state one respondent said "*we have to focus on international borders where many types of trades are being carried out. We should register the brothels and monitor it*". Political parties of the state like the congress are of the opinion of "*creating conducive environment for HIV prevention, Involvement of the church is to be encouraged*". Analysis of the responses indicates that a more reliable, transparency in services and coordination between different Ministries and participation from the local people are needed.

Of the many responses participation and owning of the issue by one and all was the felt needs of the hour.

Involvement of the politicians in media

Media, be it printed or electronics are very important modes of spreading awareness especially when there are different barriers of communication. Politicians of the state are sometimes invited by the media to talk about HIV and AIDS. Some of the responses showed that they had been invited by media to talk about HIV and AIDS. One respondent says he has already been approached by the media to talk about the issue of HIV and AIDS in various capacities. "*I was invited twice by the media as a speaker of Manipur Legislative Assembly and as president of Manipur Legislative Forum on HIV and AIDS*". One of the members has been invited on many occasions to talk about HIV and AIDS as a secretary of Manipur Legislative Forum on HIV and AIDS.

Political leaders showed their willingness to espouse and stand for the cause of HIV and AIDS mitigation in their constituency. Showing their willingness in action, members interacted and consulted the church youths and pastors to give awareness about HIV and AIDS when holding a mass. Being elected representative they made use of their status. "*Being an M.L.A I can take advantage of the crowds who gathered during a meeting and spread awareness. I mobilized the church leaders and village chiefs association within my constituency for awareness generation towards the causes of HIV and AIDS*". One of the respondent said that he has been campaigning for the removal of stigma and discrimination in the minds of the people within his constituency as and when he got any chances to speak to the people.

The involvement and the willingness of the politicians could be seen as their response show *"I will stand by the need of the people within my constituency in particular and the needs of the people from the state of Manipur in general"*. Politicians also showed their willingness to train the elected members like Zilla Parishad, Pradhans, etc so that they act as a middlemen between the MLA and the people.

Opinion on the manner of surveillance and reporting of HIV and AIDS in the state

Opinion varies regarding satisfaction level of surveillance and reporting on HIV and AIDS. The sentinel surveillance on HIV and AIDS in Manipur is being carried out by Indian Council of Medical Research (ICMR) and Regional Institute of Medical Sciences (RIMS) microbiology departments.

Few of the responses indicate that there are respondents who don't have idea about the survey citing unavailability of scientific reports. After carefully analyzing the response there at times are exaggerations by some groups of the total number of HIV positive people in the state. The responses show that the idea of having regular surveillance in a regular manner would be good.

> *"There is under or over estimation, thus surveillance should be carried out in a regular manner. Exaggeration by some NGOs should not be done and also the state government can do more intensive and use scientific technique".*

Opinion on priority issues pertaining to HIV and AIDS showed shades of opinion that prevention and its methods and strategy were given most important followed by tackling stigma, treatment and targeted intervention for specific groups like women and children. Prevention strategies should focus on reducing stigma and greater investment in treatment is needed.

ASSEMBLY BUDGET ALLOCATION AND UTILIZATION OF LOCAL AREA DEVELOPMENT FUND (LADF) FOR HIV AND AIDS

After analyzing the responses and opinions regarding assembly budget allocation, budgets for HIV and AIDS takes a backstage. Priorities were given to developmental issues like education, road construction and building of infrastructure. It has been viewed that the gravity of the HIV virus has not really reached the minds of the policy makers. Though certain amount of budget has been earmarked for HIV and AIDS the amount is not sufficient to tackle the present crisis. "*Budgets are planned according to the requirement of the state. But personally I would like to appeal to the authority to give priority to health related matters as we all know the saying "Health is Wealth",*" said one of the respondents. The government also lack priority in budget allocation for the cause of HIV and AIDS. This can be substantiated by a response given by one respondent "*It lacks priority on budget allocation but we are pressing hard to the government*".

With regard to utilization of Local Area Development Fund (LADF) for the causes of HIV and AIDS it draws a mixture of response. One of the respondents said that "*Specific guidelines are set up by the government so we cannot spend any money till now. We spoke to the Chief Minister*". Another respondent said "*certain dos' and don'ts are there on how to utilize LAD fund. HIV and AIDS was not in the list, but now they have included and we will see how*". Some of the responses showed that they have already spent certain amount of money towards the issue.

Budget allocation and the importance given with regard to HIV and AIDS can be criticized as there has never been a special session in Manipur with respect to HIV and AIDS. None of the responses also has any indication of having conducted so far.

MANIPUR ASSEMBLY PROCEDURE AND HIS EXCELLENCY THE GOVERNORS' ADDRESS ON HIV AND AIDS

The Manipur Legislative Assembly follows a unicameral system. The assembly procedure has question hour, Zero hour, call attention motion, discussion and voting on demands for grants, etc. Generally, the first hour of a sitting of the assembly is committed to questions and that hour is called the Question Hour. It has a particular significance in the proceedings of the assembly. It is during the Question Hour that the members can ask questions on every aspect of administration and Governmental activity.

A Starred Question is one to which a member desires an oral answer in the House and which is distinguished by an asterisk mark. When a question is answered orally, supplementary questions can be asked thereon.

An Unstarred Question is one which is not called for oral answer in the House and on which no supplementary questions can consequently be asked. To such a question, a written answer is deemed to have been laid on the Table after the Question Hour by the Minister to whom it is addressed. It is printed in the official report of the sitting of the House for which it is put down.

The content of the assembly proceedings has been discussed under different topic heads starting with the address made by His Excellency the governor of Manipur. During the period under consideration for analysis of assembly discussion and debates 2002-2010 there has been four successive governors' in Manipur. 1. Shri. Ved Prakash Marwah from 2nd December 1999 to 12th June 2003. 2. Shri Arvind Dave from 13th June 2003 to 5th August 2004. 3. Dr. Shivinder Singh Sidhu from 6th August 2004 to 23rd July 2008 and 4. Shri Gurbachan Jagat from 23rd July 2008 until writing of this thesis. The period 2002-2010 has been choosen keeping in mind the availability of documents to support the analysis.

Shri Ved Prakash Marwah the then governor of Manipur in his address to the 8th Manipur Legislative Assembly on 12.03.2002 said that "*The growing menace of HIV and AIDS in the State is a matter of serious concern to all of us. Up to the end of January, 2001, as many as 11,271 HIV positive cases were detected in the State. Under the AIDS Control programme being implemented with Central assistance by the Manipur AIDS Control Society, 100% screening has been introduced in all the Blood Banks in Manipur. AIDS education has been introduced in the school's curriculum from class VI to X. The AIDS Control Society has also set up 17 Targeted Intervention Projects in the six high prevalence districts of the State. A time has come to evaluate the success of the ongoing AIDS control programme and to take new initiatives to eliminate this scourge of mankind. My Govt. is committed to providing total healthcare and will take special steps for re-vitalizing the primary healthcare system in the rural areas. External aid will also be tapped for upgrading the secondary healthcare system in the State".*

The said governor of Manipur, His Excellency Shri Ved Prakash Marwah on 11-03-2003 said "*as I have mentioned earlier, the prevalence of HIV and AIDS in the State is a cause of serious concern. As many as 14,837 HIV positive cases have already been detected in Manipur. Under the AIDS Control Programme, which is being implemented by the Manipur State AIDS Control Society, cent percent screening has been introduced in the three Blood Banks namely RIMS Hospital, JN Hospital and District Hospital, Churachandpur. The Society has also set up 28 Targeted Intervention Projects in the state. Aids education curriculum has been introduced in the schools from classes IV to X. A project to carry out the feasibility study of transmission of HIV from mother to child has been started in all the districts of Manipur. It is hoped that with these measures and with the cooperation of the people, it will be possible to control the menace of AIDS in the State".*

His Excellency Shri Ved Prakash Marwah from his statement made before the elected representatives within these two consecutive years shows his commitment and his desire to control and reverse the pandemic. However in the matter of steps already taken up by the state government a response from the beneficiaries shows that the increase of targeted intervention projects from 17 to 28 was not enough to cater to the needs of the people. One notable initiative taken up by Mr Ved Prakash would be the introduction of schools AIDS education from class VI to X.

His Excellency Shri Arvind Dave the Governor of Manipur from June 2003 to 5th August 2004 on his statement to the Manipur legislative assembly on 06-02-2004 didn't particularly mention about benefits and welfare schemes for people Living With HIV and AIDS though, he talked about commitment in providing quality Health and Family Welfare services to the people in general. Besides giving emphasis on improvement and for Upgradation of medical infrastructure like increasing the number of mobile dispensary units from 3 to 6 he talked about construction of 100 bedded hospitals in thoubal district and the construction of trauma centre at Jawaharlal Nehru hospital in porompat, Imphal.

His Excellency, the governor of Manipur, Dr. Shivinder Singh Sidhu from 6th August 2004 to 23rd July 2008 address the Manipur Legislative Assembly for four consecutive years on 15-03-2005, 22-02-2006, 16-3-2007 and 1-2-2008.

During the first two years of his address to the assembly, he talked about the gravity of the issue and the steps and initiatives undertaken by Manipur state AIDS control Society in collaboration with international NGO's like Bill and Melinda gates foundation and Medicin Sans Frontiers (MSF-Doctors without borders). A project called Organized Response for Comprehensive HIV Interventions in selected High-prevalence Districts (ORCHID) was initiated in May 2004 as collaboration between Emmanuel Hospital Association (EHA) and Australian International Health Institute (AIHI), now Nossal Institute for Global Health, University of Melbourne. Project ORCHID has been working to reduce transmission of HIV and STI among Injecting Drug Users (IDUs), Female Sex Workers (FSWs), Men who have Sex with Men (MSM) and their sexual partners through a response of increased scale and coverage in selected high -prevalence districts and townships of Manipur and Nagaland in Northeast (NE) India. He said in his 2006 assembly address "*project ORCHID supplements the efforts of the State Government. Also, Medicines sans Frontiers, an International NGO based in Holland in collaboration with Manipur AIDS Control Society has started ART (anti retroviral therapy) for 500 AIDS patients in Churachandpur District*".

His Excellency Dr. Shivinder Singh sidhu in his address to the Manipur legislative assembly on 16-3-2007 said "*My Government is deeply concerned with the prevailing incidence of HIV and AIDS, a major health concern in the State today. Accordingly, the Manipur State AIDS Control Society has been implementing various programmes for prevention of the spread of HIV and AIDS. Harm reduction is integrated with care component under "Rapid Intervention and Care" (RIAC) Project. Adequate focus is given to IEC campaigns and social advocacy programmes. Anti retroviral drugs are given to the needy patients at four ART Centres at J.N.Hospital, Imphal, RIMS Imphal, District Hospital Churachandpur and District Hospital, Ukhrul.* He also in his address said that *a fifth ART Centre is being opened at District Hospital, Thoubal by the end of March 2008".*

The governor address shows commitment of the government by not only depending on international initiatives but initiatives of Indian government and the state concerned. His Excellency Dr. Shivinder Singh Sidhu on his address to Manipur legislative assembly on 1-2-2008 focussed his address to commitment in medical infrastructure of the state. He said "*my government is committed to make health care facilities accessible to all sections of the society specially the remote and the rural areas. The state, therefore, has proposed to construct one fifty (150) bedded hospital each at Ukhrul, Senapati, Tamenglong, Chandel and Jiribam. The JN Hospital is being upgraded to 300 bedded hospitals and all efforts have been made to convert this complex into Jawaharla Nehru Institute of Medical Sciences. The acquisition of land has already been made. The state is also implementing National health programmes like National vector borne disease control, National T.B Control, National leprosy control, National programme for blindness, National AIDS control and the Iodine deficiency disease programmes*". Regardless, commitment of the governor could be seen in infrastructural development for general health care in his address but particular mention was not made regarding people living with HIV and AIDS in particular and the causes of HIV and AIDS in general.

His Excellency Shri Gurbachan Jagat the governor of Manipur assumes his office on 23rd July 2008 and has been serving the state until writing of this thesis. His Excellency Shri Gurbachan Jagat gave a scientific report in his address to Manipur legislative assembly on 17-3- 2009. He appraised the state of being the first in formulating a specific HIV and AIDS policy in the country. He said "*Manipur was the first state in India to formulate a state AIDS policy in 1996. But HIV and AIDS continues to plague the state. As per NFHS-*

3, the HIV prevalence in Manipur is 1.13% as compared to an All India average of 0.36. 30446 cases of HIV have been detected till date. Recognizing the gravity of the situation, my government has taken up steps to improve the functioning of the Manipur AIDS control society (MACS). Given the alarming signs of spread of the virus to general population, I would urge one and all to undergo voluntary testing in any of the 54 integrated counseling & testing centre. Early detection would enable timely initiation of free ART in the 7 ART centers in the state". He also talked about organizing a program "*A grand function was organized at Imphal on 1st December 2008 to observe the world AIDS day wherein 2nd line ART was also launched*". He said the strategies of the government and various stake holders should involve concerted efforts from all quarters *"a joint concerted effort is vital if we are to successfully halt and reverse the spread of HIV epidemic in Manipur".*

His Excellency Shri Gurbachan Jagat the governor of Manipur in his address to Manipur legislative assembly on 13-01-2010 focused his address on the achievement of the state government. He spoke about how HIV was first detected in Manipur and the success achieved due to the HIV and AIDS policy 1996 by introducing Rapid Intervention and Care project. He said "*as honorable members would be aware that HIV transmission in Manipur originated primarily among Injecting Drug Users, especially heroin users. Accordingly, a special project titled "Rapid intervention and Care was launched in 1999-2000 with the aim of reducing HIV transmission among IDUs through the needle syringe exchange programme. Manipur was the first state in India to have adopted this strategy based on the principle of Harm reduction or Harm minimization. This pioneering intervention by Manipur State AIDS Control Society has been very successful and HIV prevalence rate among the IDU's has declined from 72.78% in 1998 to 17.9% in 2007. This is a commendable achievement".*

The then governor appraise of the achievement and initiatives of the state government saying "*Voluntary HIV testing is critical in successfully tackling of the spread of this dreadful virus. On the occasion of 2009 World AIDS Day, 5 more mobile Integrated Counseling & Testing Centre Vans were launched to provide better testing coverage in the hill districts. The number of HIV testing centres in Manipur has increased from 12 in 2005 to 54 in 2008".*

"The Manipur legislator's forum on HIV and AIDS was formed on 30th June 2007 with the objective of involving elected legislators to change the course of the pandemic of HIV and AIDS in the state. I am happy to inform that Rs. 60 lakhs has been allocated out of the MLA Local Area Development fund for use by the legislator's forum".

"With these efforts there are encouraging signs. As per latest NACO estimation, adult HIV prevalence has gone down from 1.67% in 2006 to 1.57% in 2007. The number of pregnant mother tested for HIV and found HIV positive decreased from 2.04% in 2001 to 1.3% in 2007. My government would spare no efforts in reducing and reversing the HIV prevalence in Manipur"

The four successive governors of Manipur shows commitment towards the greater causes of Health care and three governors of the period went to the extent in their address by particularly quoting causes and concerns of people living with HIV and AIDS.

DISCUSSION AND DEBATES IN THE ASSEMBLY

Discussion and debates in the assembly from 2002- 2010 has been analyzed as under to find out the realities of the representatives of the state in their commitment for the cause of HIV and AIDS. The period 2002-2010 has been chosen keeping in mind the availability of government records as explained earlier. The analysis has been done dividing them according to the issue as it appears in the assembly proceeding procedures.

Discussion and voting on demand for grants

During the period under consideration 2002-2010 under the heading discussion and voting on demands for grants, particular topics on HIV and AIDS has been discussed 10 times according to assembly proceedings of the state.

During 2010 it was only Shri Radhabinod Koijam, MLA moving cut motion during discussion and voting on demand for grants drew the attention of the minister for giving benefits to people living with HIV and AIDS and infected mothers and children

Dr. I. Ibohalbi, MLA and secretary general of Manipur legislators' forum on HIV and AIDS moving a cut motions during 2009 pointed out that Manipur health care delivery system was outdated and highlighted the need for its improvement and its proper policy to tackle infectious disease, non infectious disease and maternity & child health, etc. He also said that the Community Health Centres in the state was not provided with adequate doctors which led to the congestion of patients at Imphal and further wanted to know the number of specialist doctors at present and its requirement as well. He also suggested for a separate directorate for Public Health. He also drew attention of the Minister on the lack of doctors in the district hospitals, number of functional ART Centres in the districts, increase of AIDS patients in Bishnupur district. He also drew attention of the Minister on implementation of 25% Non Practicing Allowance (NPA) for doctors of the state, ban on government doctors practice in private hospitals, step of the government for an awareness programme to help in reducing stigma on HIV and AIDS.

Dr. Ng. Bijoy Singh, MLA moving cut motions during 2009 observed that regardless of improving health status of the state; the secondary and tertiary sector of the state lacks efficiency and also pointed out the needs for manpower development. Commenting on the need to give more emphasis on Public Health Sector he said that sufficient funds should be provided. He also talked about decentralization of school health programme which are needed for addressing the grievances of Accredited Social Health Activist (ASHA), empanelling of Shija Hospitals and CMC Koirengei and the need to maintain vital statistics of HIV patients. Highlighting the present menace of drugs, he said that effective drug control administration was required.

Shri Radhabinod Koijam, MLA moving cut motion during 2009 pointed out the huge prevalence of HIV infected persons in the state and the social hazards that such people could posed if proper attention were not paid to them and critically commented on failure of the department to pay attention to the widows and children of HIV infected persons. He urged the department to see if AAY cards, vocational training and reservation of jobs could be made available to widows and infected persons.

Shri Ph. Parijat Singh, Minister (Health and Family Welfare Services) clarifying to the demand discussion during 2009 informed that health services in the state had improved considerably with the implementation of NRHM. Mobile Medical Units were kept stationed at district hospitals after fitting the required equipment and giving services to the sick patients. He said "*For effective implementation of HIV and AIDS prevention programs the government was contemplating to constitute District AIDS Prevention and Control Units, with the DCs as the Chairman, CMOs as Vice Chairman and the MLAs, concerned, as Advisors, to all the districts and the MLAs would contribute 1 lakh each and 60 lakhs by the Government for its fund, he informed. The dead rate due to HIV infection had decreased with the opening of ART Centres providing medicines to infected persons in the state, he said, and added that 4 new Link ART Centres would be opened very soon*".

Analysis of the 2009 assembly proceedings during discussion and voting on demand for grants shows the inadequacy of the number of trained doctors especially in the hill districts of the state. There has been no specific policy and guidelines for the children, women and widows of HIV and AIDS infected persons. However the commitment of the government could be seen as new programmes are being introduced like ART link centre's in the state to cater to the needs of people especially for PLWHA.

During the year 2008 Dr. I. Ibohalbi, MLA and secretary general of Manipur legislators' forum on HIV and AIDS moving cut motions pointed out the disparity in the reports made by the Family Welfare Department and Medical &Health Department of the infant mortality rate. Regarding the lack of specialist in Government run hospitals, he wanted the Government to increase the non-practicing allowances, provide better facilities for the doctors posted in the hills and to give promotion avenues every 5 or 10 years. He expressed apprehension that the District Mobile Unit opened under the Rural Health Mission might not be able to cater its service successfully due to the poor condition of roads in hill districts. The budget allocation for Health Sub-Centers, PHCs and CHCs was made only for infrastructural development and was lacking in other areas, he said. He wanted the Government to provide ambulance facilities to PHCs, blood bank and storage facilities to District head quarters, install MRIs in the state hospitals and also to properly manage hospital waste by installing incinerators. "*He said the rate of HIV/AIDS was highest in the country and its funding was made only by National AIDS Control Society and to create a sense of belongingness and responsibility, State Government should allocate funds for it. He said that Government should adopt a new policy programming to revive the Public Health Sector Undertakings*".

During the year 2003, Shri N. Bihari Singh, MLA expressed his desires by moving a cut motion requesting the members to consent on equal distribution of funds sanctioned under AIDS Awareness Programme to all the districts of Manipur.

The year 2002 before the end of the 1st Phase of NACP was a crucial year for both the government at the centre and at the state. The leader of the opposition party of Manipur Shri O Joy and D Shaija MLA on 25th July 2002 pointed out to government of many loopholes and gaps as far as care, treatment and support services to people living with HIV and AIDS are concerned.

In reply to a particular question on Prevention of Mother to Child Transmission at Maram health centre, the health minister said that the state cabinet has approved of recruiting counselors and technicians. Delegation of work on prevention of mother to child transmission in progress has to be implemented in a smoother manner.

Shri O. Joy leader of the opposition party to Health Minister questioned about the construction of 100 bedded hospital out of the money earmarked for treatment and prevention of HIV and AIDS. In response to a question, the health minister clarified that the money was sanctioned by NACO for the said construction.

Due to the alarming situations of HIV and AIDS, all party meetings including organization's clubs and various stake holders for prevention of HIV and AIDS was convened at the governor's chamber.

Shri O Joy continued s*ince "AIDS has become one of the most serious issues pertaining to the state, the government should leave no stone unturned to combat the issue. Awareness components should be included in Leela's (Popular folk plays), Radio and television and school going children's text books".*

Shri O Joy to the health minister enquired about the much hyped HIV and AIDS bill. He also pointed out that "*certain developed countries and richer states of India have already started the campaign against HIV and AIDS by providing anti HIV drugs at free of cost to its citizens. Patients are patients whether they are Manipuri or others, then why wait?* Further he said i*s it possible to ask the poor to die as they cannot afford to pay for their prescribed drugs? It is high time for the government to look into it very seriously".*

In reply to a clarification sought by Shri O Joy, the health Minister said "*regarding the construction of a 100 bedded hospital at Porompat is true but the funds have been sanctioned by NACO. It has been constructed out of the Rs. 60 Lakh released by NACO. The project has been on halt for the moment as the remaining amount has not been released by NACO, a detailed work report has already been sent to NACO for the next release".*

The minister continues "*an intervention plan will be strategically worked out looking into the trends of HIV infection in Manipur. The main route of HIV infection in the country is through sexual routes but in the states of Manipur it ismainly through intravenous drug users".*

Showing commitment of his government, the health minister said "*Manipur is the first and only state in India having a clear cut HIV and AIDS policy since 1996 till now. No other states of India have such policy document so far. The Manipur state AIDS control society (MSACS) has introduced an innovative project for the year covering 200 people and whatever work has been carried out no other states in India had earlier initiated".*

"At present the number of AIDS patient is 1876 as reported by MSACS. A total number of 1302 confirmed cases of AIDS had died since the first case was reported in Manipur. Medical experts has pointed out that there would be more than 100 deaths due to HIV/AIDS but they were not properly diagnosed or examined for HIV and AIDS".

"Above all we should find a way on how to prevent ourselves and as suggested by the member steps would be taken up to include in various forms of communications suggested for the general population".

Shri O. Joy continuing the discussion pointed out that the Leela (Folk Drama) which has been prescribed by the health minister contains an explicit illicit material, but not suitable for the societal viewership. In reply to the query the minister said that "*the real intentions of the Leela's party were to give clear cut information about the intricacies on HIV and AIDS. They might have played it several times overlooking the limits of it. I myself will look into the matter*".

Shri O. Joy to the health minister about providing ART facility in the state, the later said "*it is very true that the said drugs cannot cure the patient but prevent the virus from progression. Few other countries and states have already introduced the drugs and in Manipur some of the positive patients have already started using the drugs. Due to high cost of the drugs it is not affordable to all though it has come down gradually. Now the real challenge is on how to introduce in the state at subsidized rate which otherwise the state is deprived of economic prosperity due to various reasons*".

Zero Hour

There have been two instances where member of the assembly raised question during zero hour about HIV and AIDS within the stated period 2002-2010. On 13th March, 2006 Shri I. Hemochandra Singh, MLA drew the attention of the Medical Minister on the irregularities while appointing Procurement Officer in Manipur AIDS Control Society (MACS). He expressed that necessary Departmental Promotion Committees (DPCs) should be conducted in the interest of the public.

Again on 22nd July, 2009 Shri Th. Shyamkumar Singh, MLA raised a query regarding the facilities provided by government for prevention of mother to child transmission of HIV.

Analysis of the nature of query and response shows that one of the queries has been of policy related matters as it concerned with recruitment policies and another relates to programming on HIV and AIDS.

Discussion on the motion of thanks to the governor's address

The governor's address has been commented twice during the stated period 2002-2010. The comment shows the requirement of a specific policy on HIV and AIDS though the state has one. However the comment signifies that some part of the policy needed amendment. To substantiate the argument on 24th February, 2006 Shri L. Ibomcha Singh, MLA moving amendment to the Motion of Thanks to the Governor's Address said that "*a specific policy was required to control HIV and AIDS*".

On 23rd February, 2006 Dr. S. Budhichandra, MLA seconder of the Motion of Thanks to the Governor's Address tried to show the government commitment by saying that "*the Government had been trying to solve the acute problem of HIV and AIDS and also to establish Rehabilitation Centre's with external fund, he added*".

Consideration and passing of government bills

In the pretext of consideration and passing of government bills the nature of discussion indicates the mismanagement of government funds regarding HIV and AIDS. In the august house on 18th July, 2005 Shri O. Joy Singh, MLA observed that the plan allocation for Manipur was not adequate. He requested Health Minister to clarify on the alleged misuse of AIDS fund.

On 17th March, 2006 Shri M. Bhorot Singh, MLA participating in the consideration, expressed suspicion of financial mismanagement, particularly the fund forwarded by the National AIDS Control Society to Manipur AIDS Control Society.

Private Members' Resolution

There has been only one occasion within the period of study 2002-2010 that a member moved a private resolution. However the move exemplifies how serious the members of the assembly are on HIV and AIDS cases. On Friday the 18th March, 2005 Shri B.D. Behring, MLA moved a Private Members' Resolution to make necessary rule/ law to conduct ELISA test on both boys and girls before marriage. He expressed his concerns over the alarming increase of HIV and AIDS infected persons in the state and added that a law should be made to insure compulsory HIV testing before marriage. He wanted the government to provide such testing facilities to all health centers within the state. In reply to the motion moved by Shri B.D Behring, Shri L. Nandakumar Singh, Minister (Health) replying to the discussion said that "*it would be difficult to legislate a law for compulsory HIV test because of various ramifications which could be counterproductive. He assured the House that testing facilities besides J.N. Hospital and RIMS would be provided to the health centers of other districts*"

DISCUSSION

Political commitment as discussed been viewed according to a model developed by Johnson 1999 that specifies three basic types of commitment a) Structural commitment b) Personal and c) Moral.

Structural Commitment

It has been viewed according to the availability of ARV Drugs and Alternative drugs like generic medicine, Investment in physical set up for Care, Support and Treatment services, Promotion of Research and Development, etc. It also looks into State commitment through continued support for local mitigation planning, State legislation enacting laws for supports, States commitment through state funding and strengthening the health care system.

As has been highlighted ARV drugs are being provided in two major hospital at the capital and various district hospitals of the state. His Excellency the Governor's address on physical infrastructure (Assembly proceedings Vol.72 Appendix A18) shows the government commitment on HIV/AIDS mitigation Care, Support and Treatment services and Promotion of Research and Development, etc. The launching of Manipur state AIDS policy and subsequent revision and adoption by the state Legislative Assembly showed political commitment on enactment of laws and policy for HIV/ AIDS Mitigation. With regard to allocation of budget and funding the elected representatives are required to donate Rs. 100,000 (One lakhs only) to the Legislative Forum on HIV/AIDS. Furthermore flexibility has been provided to elected representatives that they can use Local Area Development Fund for HIV/AIDS mitigation programmes. The up-gradation of Jawaharlal Nehru Hospital, Regional Institute of Medical Sciences (RIMS) and various districts hospital shows political commitment through strengthening the health care system of the state.

Personal commitment

It has been viewed according to politicians attitudes towards PLWHA, Personal promises made if any and results and Support of any HIV mitigation programme. Analysis of the responses and assembly debates shows that all the politicians are in favour of creating a Conducive environment for PLWHA for their Care, Support and Treatment services. The allocation of certain amount of money from their LADF and their interest and participation in any HIV/AIDS mitigation programmes shows their commitment.

Moral commitment

It has been viewed according to politician's sense of moral obligation towards PLWHA and the importance level of moral values accorded to the issues. Each of the politicians interviewed showed moral commitment by highlighting the need to protect the rights of PLWHA.

Commitment of the politicians in terms of providing services, infrastructure and frequency of the issues rose in the assembly debates and their involvement in various activities; forums created for HIV/ AIDS mitigation cannot be neglected. It can be concluded that on the part of the government efforts has been made and it is thus the collective responsibility of the government and various stake holders. It is difficult to come to any hard conclusions that politicians are really committed to HIV/AIDS mitigation in the state as stated earlier. Commitment is multidimensional and therefore, cannot be measured through a single quantitative indicator.

CHAPTER 6

Recommendations and Conclusion

This chapter has been divided into six (6) Parts. The first part will discuss about the existing HIV Policies, Programmes and Strategies in Manipur and will be followed by conclusion and recommendation. The second part will analyze the modalities of program implementation by the Government and Non-Governmental Organisations. The third part will try to understand the political commitment of political leaders in HIV/AIDS mitigation. The fourth part study beneficiaries perception of services rendered by Government and Non-Governmental Organisations. The fifth part discusses about major findings. Sixth Part suggests the role of professional social workers in implementing prevention, care and support programmes in the field of HIV/AIDS. Part Seven discuss about further scope of research in the topic. Part eight discuss about implication for social work practice and Part nine is the conclusion.

PART I EXISTING HIV POLICIES, PROGRAMMES AND STRATEGIES IN MANIPUR

Policies, Programmes and Strategies from the United States, European Union, African countries to South east Asian countries talks about unfettered services regardless of age, gender, race/

ethnicity, sexual orientation, gender identity or socio-economic circumstance, which will have unfettered access to high quality, life-extending care, free from stigma and discrimination. Notably United States could be commended of their commitment towards people living with HIV/AIDS prevention, care and after care services which other countries focussed mostly on prevention. The European Commission gave priority to policies on political commitment of European Countries and involvement of various civil societies, stakeholders not only on policy formulation but also on program monitoring and implementation. The commission could well be praised of their commitment in funding for NGO's and private sector cooperation. South African countries could be praised for integration of sexual and reproductive health, easy access to relevant information, bottom up governance, accountability, transparency and meaningful involvement of PLHA, effective communication, monitoring and evaluation and dedicated research has been attributed for their success. Jamaican success of the policy is based on the guiding principles of Political commitment, Transparency, accountability, Multisectoral approach and partnership, participation and protection of PLHA.

The Thailand optimization and consolidation of mother to child transmission, condom programming, prevention among the young and the youths, blood safety, stigma and discrimination and its success is due to its government commitment and the ability to create a sense of ownership to all its citizens even to the local level who are unreached otherwise. Asian countries success can be attributed to government giving prioritised interventions to control the epidemic in injection drug users, sex workers, men who have sex with men, harm minimization and additionally focuses on primary and secondary prevention, providing an enabling environment, redressing health inequities, ensuring effectiveness in achieving health outcomes, promoting good practice, etc.

In the Indian context the 1st NACP was focused on mass campaign on awareness and 2nd NACP has undergone dramatic changes focusing on prevention intervention among targeted populations, institutional strengthening and inter sectoral collaboration. Likewise the main focus of the 3rd NACP was halting and reversing the HIV/AIDS epidemic following the strategy of unified three ones, one agreed action framework, one national HIV/ AIDS coordinating authority and one agreed national M&E system. The 4th NACP aims to accelerate the process of reversal and further strengthen the epidemic response in India through a cautious and well defined integration process over the next five years. It continues to give emphasis on Unified three ones with additionally focusing on quality, innovation and integration, partnership with comprehensive care, support and treatment.

In the context of the present study Manipur for combating the menace of HIV and AIDS in Manipur, Manipur State AIDS Policy 1996 was launched focusing on various dimensions in line with NACP. Certain Positive development in the new revised Manipur State AIDS policy 1996 includes: Manipur state government will now allow utilization of MLA Local area Development Program (MLA LADP) fund; Introduction of District AIDS Prevention Control Unit (DAPCU); Inclusion of one male and female PLWHA in MSACS Committees; Policy for involvement of CBO, FBO, Social Organization only for IEC Programs; Compulsory training for student for two days to be eligible to appear for Xth and XIIth exam and teacher for three days to enter into state service; Provision of free travel for PLWHA; Provision of Opportunistic Infection drugs; Monitoring and Evaluation once in every year.

Though the state has formulated an ambitious policy on HIV and AIDS, various aspects of the policy are not fulfilled. Responses from the beneficiaries also shows that the policy didn't reach the hills people. Mention can be made that the components of compulsory training for student for two days to be eligible to appear for Xth and XIIth exam and teacher for three days to enter into state service; Provision of free travel for PLWHA; Provision of Opportunistic Infection drugs are also not implemented. Policy for involvement of CBO, FBO and Social Organizations though finds its place, there has not been any invitation to these said organization from the policy makers as responded by heads of theses organization.

PART II MODALITIES OF PROGRAM IMPLEMENTATION BY THE GOVERNMENT AND NON-GOVERNMENTAL ORGANISATIONS

This part will analyze the second objective of analyzing the modalities of program implementation by the Government and Non-Governmental Organisations.

The first initiative of the Government of India to take up the causes of HIV and AIDS was the setting up of National AIDS Control Program (NACP) in India in 1987. There has been four successive AIDS control programme. NACP I - 1992-97-99, NACP II -1999-2004-06-07, NACP III 2007-12, NACP IV-2012-17. Various strategies and action plans of the government have been discussed earlier in part I and the preceding chapters also.

Some of the main objectives of the 12 NGO's as justified in chapter IV includes: Outreach work to different communities, HIV and AIDS awareness program, condom promotion, Needle and syringe exchange program, Home based care, referral services, DOT service at drop in centre, Coordination between various positive people, Advocacy, Helping children orphaned by HIV and AIDS, SHG formation for PLWHA, Women Empowerment, eradication of illiteracy by taking up various educational programmes, HIV and AIDS intervention programmes among C.S.W, IDU, MSM, developing a strategies for effective implementation of child rights especially of HIV and AIDS infected and affected etc. Some of the main strategies adopted by NGOs in HIV and AIDS mitigation interventions are peer-group approach, capacity building of the project personnel, condom promotion strategies, accessibility of IEC materials, STD diagnosis and treatment, outreach work strategies and intervention at the community levels.

In Manipur under MSACS Rapid Intervention and Care program (RIAC), Drug rehabilitation programs, Men who has Sex with Men program (MSM Program), Needles and Syringes Exchange Programs (NSEP), etc are carried out by NGO's. The impetus for the creation and maintenance of Needle and Syringe Exchange Program (NSEP) emerged from the philosophy of harm reduction, an approach that assumes the probability of contracting or spreading HIV and AIDS is minimized by providing IDUs with clean needles at little or no cost. The concept of Harm Minimization and NSEP is a big success in the state as the number of infection due to infected Needles and Syringes has come down drastically (MSACS). Of the total respondent 38.5% reported the use of folk media in reaching out to the people. Another 23.1% felt that peer education also to be one of the most successful among the many intervention programs. Over 61.5% felt that HIV and AIDS awareness programmes in the communities seem to be the most effective of all prevention programmes while some respondents said peer education is a successful intervention strategy in their organization.

Problems like frequent Bandhs and blockages called by various organizations irrespective of social, cultural, student and political fuelled by stigma and discrimination also create a great hindrance in HIV and AIDS intervention programmes that being carried out by various organizations.

As far as funding is concern 4 organizations received from foreign donors like Catholic Relief Services, Child Rights and You, Clinton Foundation and Childline and responses showed that they are more flexible than government funding. Irregularity of the funds being released by the state government also hampers the continuity of the intervention programmes.

Services provided by the non-governmental organizations includes financial support for ration or clothes

, vocational training to PLWHA, assistance in job placement, self help group formation, educational support for children affected or infected by HIV and AIDS, facilitate formation of PLWHA network and research work and the beneficiaries are contend with. However NGO's are not having social marketing programs of condoms which otherwise has been proven successful in Thailand. Of the total respondent 23.3% are not happy with services provided by the government while another 76.7% are content with service provided by government. Another 95% are happy with the services they received from NGO. Stigma and discrimination still exist though in minimal cases.

Social and cultural organization plays an important role in tackling HIV/AIDS. India being a culturally diverse country, having strong cultural ethics, norms and values, it can go a long way in the prevention of HIV and AIDS by making use of these cultural organizations.

There are two such organizations that indirectly help in containment of HIV/AIDS. All Manipur Anti Drugs Association and Meira Paibi's (Women Torch Bearer) who are spearheading anti drugs campaign in the state. These two organizations have almost the same objective of drugs free life. However Meira Paibi's is one such organization whose presence is incomparable as they are present in each and every locality of Manipur. Considering the work and achievement of these organisations, it is important to identify, engage and increase the capacity of community support structures to support young people on drug prevention behavior. The government should engage different law and policy instruments to support youth prevention initiatives on drug abuse. The government and various social organizations in Manipur should come together and foster networking among all the likes of social Organizations.

The role of faith based organization in the mitigation of HIV/AIDS is huge as also shown in the present study. The greatest contribution of FBO's according to various faith leaders would have been the changes which are visible among clients, changes in the behavior and risk perception among the church leaders and the beneficiaries. Of the four FBO's two of them totally abhor the idea of condom promotion, they stick to the classical idea of total abstinence. The other two despite not totally detesting the idea spoke about having safer sex practices and to be patient until marriage. They do not openly distribute condoms but spoke about it directly or indirectly withholding the importance of it in the prevention of HIV and AIDS.

Study conducted within the aforesaid four FBO's whose approach to behavior change is through holistic counseling, it shows that behavior changes through these counseling has minimal cases of relapse than detoxification/ substitution model where the cases of relapse cases sky rocketed. Looking into the success and achievement of FBO's in the state of Manipur the state government through its various agencies can identify certain FBO's who are really doing well in their own part despite the size of the organization and fund their project so that the HIV sero-prevalence rate is reversed.

PART III POLITICAL COMMITMENT OF POLITICAL LEADERS IN HIV/AIDS MITIGATION

In this part political commitment has been measured indirectly by examining the statements, policies, and actions of leaders, what they have talked about HIV and AIDS or by what they actually do in varying degrees. It was seen that leaders who spoke out publicly about the importance of HIV and AIDS are expressing a commitment to the issue and creating a climate that encourages solutions.

Four of the successive governor's talked about the government commitment through Infrastructural, Institutional investment and personal commitment during the study period. As in one of the governor's address "My government is now giving special emphasis to strengthening of medical infrastructure by sourcing additional funds from (Department for the development of the north eastern region (DoNER) and North eastern Council) NEC". The successive governors of Manipur shows commitment towards the greater causes of Health care and three governors of the period went to the extent in their address by particularly quoting causes and concerns of people living with HIV and AIDS.

The formation of Manipur State Legislative Forum on HIV and AIDS (MLFA) and a series of political conventions, the declaration of Antyodaya Anna Yojana popularly known as AAY to be made available to all people living with HIV and AIDS (PLHA), etc. also shows the government commitment.

Political parties and their leaders of the state consider HIV and AIDS as a political issue as many of the response reflected it. Some of the responses went to the extent that "*it is not only political; rather it is also a social issue*". "*Yes AIDS is a political issue as politics involves human issues so HIV is directly or indirectly related to HIV and AIDS*". The involvement of different ministries other than Health and Family welfare like education, sports, transport and communication, etc. and the opinion of creating conducive environment for HIV prevention, involvement of the church, etc.

also showed commitment of the government. However analysis of the responses indicates that a more reliable, transparency in services and coordination between different Ministries and participation from the local people are needed.

Of the many responses participation and owning of the issue by one and all was the felt needs of the hour.

Opinion on priority issues pertaining to HIV and AIDS showed shades of opinion that prevention and its methods and strategy were given most important followed by tackling stigma, treatment and targeted intervention for specific groups like women and children. After analyzing the responses and opinions regarding assembly budget allocation, budgets for HIV and AIDS takes a backstage. Priorities were given to developmental issues like education, road construction and building of infrastructure. It has been viewed that the gravity of the HIV virus has not really reached the minds of the policy makers. Budget allocation and the importance given with regard to HIV and AIDS can be criticized as there has never been a special session in Manipur with respect to HIV and AIDS.

Content analysis on discussion and debates in the assembly from 2002- 2010 has been made to find out the realities of the representatives of the state in their commitment for the cause of HIV and AIDS. The period 2002-2010 has been chosen keeping in mind the availability of government records as explained earlier.

Under the heading discussion and voting on demands for grants, particular topics on HIV and AIDS have been discussed 10 times according to assembly proceedings of the state. The discussion varies from giving benefits to people living with HIV and AIDS and infected mothers and children. Up gradation of Manipur health care delivery system which was quoted as outdated and highlighted the need for its improvement and its proper policy to tackle infectious disease, non infectious disease and maternity & child health, improving health status of the state, the secondary and tertiary sector which also lacks efficiency and also pointed out the needs for manpower development. They also urged if AAY cards, vocational training and reservation of jobs could be made available to widows and infected persons. Shri Ph. Parijat Singh, Minister (Health and Family Welfare Services) said "*For effective implementation of HIV and AIDS prevention programs the government was contemplating to constitute District AIDS Prevention and Control Units, with the DCs as the Chairman, CMOs as Vice Chairman and the MLAs, concerned, as Advisors, to all the districts and the MLAs would contribute 1 lakh each and 60 lakhs by the Government for its fund, he informed. The dead rate due to HIV infection had decreased with the opening of ART Centres providing medicines to infected persons in the state, he said, and added that 4 new Link ART Centres would be opened very soon*".

Analysis of the 2009 assembly proceedings during discussion and voting on demand for grants shows the inadequacy of the number of trained doctors especially in the hill districts of the state. There has been no specific policy and guidelines for the children, women and widows of HIV and AIDS infected persons. However the commitment of the government could be seen as new programmes are being introduced like ART link centre's in the state to cater to the needs of people especially for PLWHA.

There have been two instances where member of the assembly raised question during zero hour. The question ranges from appointing Procurement Officer in Manipur State AIDS Control Society (MSACS) and facilities provided by government for Prevention of Mother to Child Transmission of HIV. Analysis of the nature of query and response shows that one of the queries has been of policy related matters as it concerned with recruitment policies and another relates to programming on HIV and AIDS.

During discussion on the motion of thanks to the governor's address there have been two instances for moving amendment to the Governor's Address which said that "*a specific policy was required to control HIV and AIDS*". While the seconder of the motion of thanks to the Governor's address tried to show the government commitment by saying that "*the Government had been trying to solve the acute problem of HIV and AIDS and also to establish rehabilitation centre's with external fund*".

In the pretext of consideration and passing of government bills the nature of discussion indicates the mismanagement of government funds regarding HIV and AIDS. One respondent participating in the consideration, expressed suspicion of financial mismanagement, particularly the fund forwarded by the National AIDS Control Society to Manipur AIDS Control Society.

There has been only one occasion within the period of study 2002-2010 that a member moved a private resolution. However the move exemplifies how serious the members of the assembly are on HIV and AIDS cases. On respondent moved a private members' resolution to make necessary rule/ law to conduct ELISA test on both boys and girls before marriage.

Political commitment as discussed been viewed according to a model developed by Johnson 1999 that specifies three basic types of commitment a) Structural commitment b) Personal and c) Moral. His Excellency the Governor's address on physical infrastructure (Assembly proceedings Vol.72 Appendix A18) shows the government commitment on HIV/AIDS mitigation Care, Support and Treatment services and Promotion of Research and Development, etc. Analysis of the responses and assembly debates shows that all the politicians are in favour of creating a Conducive environment for PLWHA for their Care, Support and Treatment services. The allocation of certain amount of money from their LADF and their interest and participation in any HIV/AIDS mitigation programmes shows their commitment. Each of the politicians interviewed showed moral commitment by highlighting the need to protect the rights of PLWHA. It can be concluded that on the part of the government efforts has been made and it is thus the collective responsibility of the government and various stake holders. It is difficult to come to any hard conclusions that politicians are really committed to HIV/AIDS mitigation in the state as stated earlier. Commitment is multidimensional and therefore, cannot be measured through a single quantitative indicator.

PART IV BENEFICIARIES PERCEPTION OF SERVICES RENDERED BY GOVERNMENT AND NON-GOVERNMENTAL ORGANISATIONS

As has been justified in the study and methodology a total of sixty (60) respondents have been selected who are all sero positive. In Manipur the incidence of HIV infection has reportedly been shifted from Intravenous Drug Users (IDU's) to the general population. The present study covering 12 Non- Governmental Organizations (NGO's) was conducted in and around Imphal east and west districts. This part analyzes beneficiaries' perception of services rendered by Government and Non-Governmental Organisations.

In the present study the age group 21-25 represents the most sexually active group among the respondents comprising 45% of the total respondents. The second highest group is 15-20 and form 16.67% of the total respondents. The ratio of male and female educational attainment is 3:4, 18:7, 7:6, 11:3 and 1:0 for primary, secondary, hr. Secondary, graduate and postgraduate respectively. There indeed is a relationship between the level of education and the HIV positivity rate amongst the respondents. Those whose educations are till secondary has the highest number of HIV positivity rate 41.67%. People who studied up to secondary level has positivity rate of 21.67% and the second highest 23.33% is in the group of respondents who studied up to graduation level. The higher the level of education is the lower the rate of HIV positivity as there is only 1.67% of positivity at the post graduation level.

Among the 60 respondents, the mean age of marriage is 25.38. The mean age of the spouse is 31.52 with the minimum of 16 and maximum age of the spouse 64. The mean number of years married is 8.78 years. The minimum number of years the respondents are married is 2years and the maximum is 22. Among the respondents, there are HIV positive couples who properly monitor and maintain their health. These types of people are longer married and lived a healthy life as compared to others who do not maintain their health. Among the respondents 28 have children and the majority of the respondents have 1 or 2 child only. 42.85% has 2 children followed by 35.71% have 1 child only. The respondent have a mean salary of Rs. 4186.67/- with minimum salary of Rs. 1500/- and maximum salary of Rs. 8000/. Among the beneficiaries not a single respondent could save a part of their earnings as they have to cough up with the rising prices whether in medicos or in their daily needs.

Personal history of the beneficiaries has been discussed in a sequential order. First it discussed about understanding the knowledge level of the beneficiaries on HIV/AIDS and their risk perception on it. Second it looked into the history of Drug use and linkages to HIV/AIDS. Thirdly it discussed about sexual history and finally on their medical history.

Knowledge level on the technicalities and the how and why of HIV infections also varies amongst the respondents. Many of the respondents do not perceive that they are at risk of infections. They consider people will have infections only if they are involved in an activity as described to be the means of HIV infection. Acceptance level and awareness on HIV and AIDS increased manifold but people still lack in-depth knowledge of HIV and AIDS. Almost half of the study population was worried about becoming infected with HIV, but only 7% were aware of their own personal vulnerability. The general perceptions, beliefs, knowledge, behavior and attitudes of the respondent differ according to their level of education in the present study group. Those with higher educational level fair better than those with lower level of education.

The mean age of Injection drug use is 23.59. There are different types of drugs used by the respondents. Most of the respondent uses drug more than once in a day, 45% of the respondents' uses thrice in a day, 32.5% use four times in a day, 15% use twice in a day. 2.5% only once and 2.5% above four times in a day. Another 5% use drugs as when they have money to get the stuff. Among the total respondents 25% uses condom every time they had sexual intercourse, 5% says they usually use quite often, 8.33% says they use sometimes when it is readily available. Out of the total 16.7% of the total says they have visited and had sexual experience with the commercial sex workers

A gender difference in the uptake of HIV testing shows that men and women testing patterns are not consistent. 20 women and 40 men who goes for blood testing and all the 20 women and 40 men are diagnosed HIV positive. The exact rate of positivity cannot be either concluded and say that positivity rates are higher among women who got tested for HIV infection or their men counterpart.

Over 75% of the total respondents received counseling services through NGO's. Majority of the NGO's used referral services as many of the NGO's are interlinked together. Treatment, prevention and after care services are very popular among the different NGO's working in the field of HIV and AIDS. Out of the total respondents n=60, 40% of the respondents received the said services. Drug detoxification program takes a new shape and was very successful in the context of Manipur as the presence of HIV among Intravenous drug users came down drastically after the inception of the program. Out of the total respondents 61.67% utilized the services of drug detoxification services being provided by the non-governmental organization. Needle and Syringe Exchange Program (NSEP) is a big hit among the NGO's who are working on Intravenous drug users. In spite of the success in NSEP there are many difficulties in the implementation. When interacted with the respondents who are receiving NSEP services in the NGO's they have many complaints about the program. Many of the respondents complained that the law enforcing agencies sometimes harassed them, when they carry used Syringes. In NSEP, clients are required to submit the used Syringes in exchange for the fresh ones. Many clients say that, the law enforcing agencies are taking advantage of people who carry used Syringes and charge them some money in order to avoid unnecessary detention. Out of the total respondents 83.33% said they receive fresh Needle and Syringes regularly. As far as ART is concern a total of n=60 were asked on whether they receive ART regularly from the government, 100% say they received it regularly. Out of the total respondents 81.7% say that their level of understanding about prevention (T.I, STI Care, ICTC, Blood Safety, IEC, Condom promotion) is good and 18.3% says that their level of understanding is fair. As far as Care (Treatment of O.I, Provision of free DOT treatments, PEP, ART) is concern 28.3% and 71.7% says that their level of understanding is good and fair respectively. A total of 11.7% and 88.3% of the respondents say that their understanding about collaboration is good and fair respectively. A total of n=60 respondents were asked on their level of understanding about capacity building (Programme management, AIDS vaccine initiative, M&E etc.) and 5% and 95% of the respondents say that their understanding level is good and fair respectively.

There is a need to decriminalize sex work and drug use if injecting drug users and sex workers are to receive and access the care they need. Responding to demands for more equitable access to care is integral to creating broad, demand driven strategies that respond to the desire by households and communities to protect themselves from HIV and its effects. Demand driven HIV prevention is likely to succeed far more readily than supply driven approaches. Also addressing the economic, political, social and cultural factors that render individuals and communities vulnerable to HIV/AIDS is crucial to a sustainable and expanded international, National and Regional response.

It can be concluded that the respondents are happy with the services provided by the government and NGO's except for negligible number of respondents wanted government to provide drugs for opportunistic infections and subsidized the rates of basic necessities for people living with HIV and AIDS.

PART V. MAJOR FINDINGS

- Policies, Programmes and Strategies from the United States, European Union, African countries to South east Asian countries talks about unfettered services regardless of age, gender, race/ethnicity, sexual orientation, gender identity or socio-economic circumstance, which will have unfettered access to high quality, life-extending care, free from stigma and discrimination.
- Though the state of Manipur has formulated an ambitious policy on HIV and AIDS, various aspects of the policy are not fulfilled.
- The policy didn't reach the hills people. Mention can be made that the components of compulsory training for student for two days to be eligible to appear for Xth and XIIth exam and teacher for three days to enter into state service; Provision of free travel for PLWHA; Provision of Opportunistic Infection drugs are also not implemented.
- Policy for involvement of CBO, FBO and Social Organizations though finds its place, there has not been any invitation to these said organization from the policy makers as responded by heads of theses organization.

- Faith based leaders does not openly support the idea of condom promotion but promote the responsible use of it for protection from various diseases.
- The government and various social organizations in Manipur should come together and foster networking among all the likes of social Organizations.
- FBO's approach to behaviour change through holistic counselling, shows that behaviour changes through these counselling has minimal cases of relapse than detoxification/ substitution model where the cases of relapse cases sky rocketed.
- Looking into the success and achievement of FBO's in the state of Manipur the state government through its various agencies can identify certain FBO's who are really doing well in their own part despite the size of the organization and fund their project so that the HIV sero-prevalence rate is reversed.
- Political leaders who spoke out publicly about the importance of HIV and AIDS are expressing a commitment to the issue and creating a climate that encourages solutions.
- Analysis of the responses and assembly debates shows that all the politicians are in favour of creating a Conducive environment for PLWHA for their Care, Support and Treatment services.
- The allocation of certain amount of money from LADF and their interest and participation in any HIV/AIDS mitigation programmes shows their commitment.
- Each of the politicians interviewed showed moral commitment by highlighting the need to protect the rights of PLWHA.
- On the part of the government efforts has been made and it is thus the collective responsibility of the government and various stake holders. It is difficult to come to any hard conclusions that politicians are really committed to HIV/

AIDS mitigation in the state as stated earlier. Commitment is multidimensional and therefore, cannot be measured through a single quantitative indicator.

- The respondents are happy with the services provided by the government and NGO's except for negligible number of respondents wanted government to provide drugs for opportunistic Infections and subsidized the rates of basic necessities for people living with HIV and AIDS.
- The concept of Harm Minimization and NSEP is a big success in the state as the number of infection due to infected Needles and Syringes has come down drastically
- HIV and AIDS awareness programmes in the communities seem to be the most effective of all prevention programmes.
- Irregularity of the funds being released by the state government hampers the continuity of the intervention programmes.
- The age group 21-25 represents the most sexually active group among the respondents
- There indeed is a relationship between the level of education and the HIV positivity rate amongst the respondents. The higher the level of education is the lower the rate of HIV positivity.
- The general perceptions, beliefs, knowledge, behaviour and attitudes of the respondent differ according to their level of education in the present study group. Those with higher educational level fair better than those with lower level of education.
- HIV positive couples who properly monitor and maintain their health are longer married and lived a healthy life as compared to others who do not maintain their health
- Needle and Syringe Exchange Program (NSEP) is a big success among the NGO's who are working for Intravenous drug users

- Law enforcing agencies are taking advantage of a person who carries used Syringe and charges them some money in order to avoid unnecessary detention.
- There is a need to decriminalize sex work and drug use if injecting drug users and sex workers are to receive and access the care they need.
- Demand driven HIV prevention is likely to succeed far more readily than supply driven approaches. Also addressing the economic, political, social and cultural factors that render individuals and communities vulnerable to HIV/AIDS is crucial to a sustainable and expanded international, national and Regional response.

PART VI ROLE OF PROFESSIONAL SOCIAL WORKERS

Roles of professional social workers have been taken from professional social workers working in organization as functionaries. There are only five professional social workers among the 24 functionaries working in the 12 organization. Suggestion ranges from working at the grassroots level, conducting research, providing counseling services, understanding the current issues, policy framing/ making partners and overall acting as advisor in programme planning and implementation. Thus social work can focus in these areas by applying different social work methods that include social case work to have an in-depth understanding about the individual's psycho-social-economic problems for intervention. Social group work method can be applied for group discussion among network of positive people where they would share without hesitation their negative and positive experiences which can be capitalize for program planning and implementation. Community organization method can be used for spreading awareness about HIV/AIDS, selection of sample and the universe for programme planning and intervention. Social welfare administration method will be useful as many of the organization under study are not well administered. Social research method will be useful to understand the gravity of the situation, policy framing and changes, etc. Social action as a method will be useful to propagate or lobby the government or policy makers for the rights of PHLA.

Some of their suggestions in details: As a professional social worker one need to know the ups and downs of the work, besides the knowledge of HIV/AIDS; one should be very committed to the program of action; work as service provider to the community; As a leader one need to lead the team members in the programme planning and action taken; Motivate the people, encourage them, plan in advance ones' program and manage the project efficiently; Proper follow up services, operational research and studying and understanding the people at the grass root level; One can take active part in counselling and give care and support services to the people as they are professionally trained also can play a responsible role in counselling and dealing with the family's problems and since one has proper understanding of the current issues he can act as advisor in programme planning and implementation.

PART VII FURTHER SCOPE OF RESEARCH

After carefully studying and analyzing policies, programmes and strategies and the role of social cultural organization few gaps have been identified for further research and studies.

1. HIV Policies and its impact on People Living with HIV/AIDS.
2. Relationship between sex work, drug use, insurgency and HIV/AIDS
3. In-depth studies on stigma and discrimination on HIV/AIDS and its reality.
4. Traditional and religious leaders' contribution in HIV/AIDS mitigation at community level.

It is hope that the findings of the present study would contribute its mite to the policy makers and contribute for the welfare of People Living with HIV/AIDS.

PART VIII IMPLICATION FOR SOCIAL WORK PRACTICE

The key findings of the present study demonstrate the relevance of structural social work perspective in HIV/AIDS prevention, control, care and support activities. More specifically, the findings of the study identified the crucial need for holistic social work practice. There are two fold goals for structural social work. First, it alleviates negative effects of structural exploitation on the people; and second, simultaneously transforms the social structure through social reforms and social change initiatives. The findings and observation of the present study is significant for current social work practice. Specifically the main routes of HIV transmission in Manipur is through Intravenous drug users and the present study correspond to using holistic approach through structural social work practice. People who use drugs are often engaged with helping professionals, including social workers and social service workers. There is a clear need for social workers and social service workers to have the support of their governing agencies to serve all of their clients, free from a prohibitionist, judgmental stance. Social work core values mirror those of harm reduction; they recognize the inherent worth and dignity of all people, take a non-judgmental stance, respect diverse populations, encourage professional competency and the right to self-determination, advocate for social justice, adopt a strengths perspective, encourage ongoing research and evaluation, and facilitate inter-professional practice. There is a lack of guidelines within social work and social service work, which is identified as a major concern in the realm of harm reduction practice. The need for harm reduction practices within social work and social service work is further evidenced by the correlation between injection drug use and HIV and Hepatitis C transmission. Incorporating harm reduction practices, values and supportive guidelines in social work will effectively reduce the negative health and social burdens on people who use drugs.

The findings of the study also suggest relevance of critical approach to social work research. As critical research discovers myths and empowers people to change their circumstances; It works from theory that most individual and institutional relationships are based on conflict and hidden structures; It theorizes that people have unrealized potential and it contends that false beliefs hide true power. It helps people see how to build a better world; It unveils illusions caused by scarce resources and it states that all science involves values, some right, some not.

PART IX CONCLUSION

Policies, Programmes and Strategies from the United States, European Union, African countries to South east Asian countries talks about unfettered services regardless of age, gender, race/ ethnicity, sexual orientation, gender identity or socio-economic circumstance, which will have unfettered access to high quality, life-extending care, free from stigma and discrimination.

Though the state of Manipur has formulated an ambitious policy on HIV and AIDS, various aspects of the policy are not fulfilled. Responses from the beneficiaries also shows that the policy didn't reach the hills people. Mention can be made that the components of compulsory training for student for two days to be eligible to appear for Xth and XIIth exam and teacher for three days to enter into state service; Provision of free travel for PLWHA; Provision of Opportunistic Infection drugs are also not implemented. Policy for involvement of CBO, FBO and Social Organizations though finds its place, there has not been any invitation to these said organization from the policy makers as responded by heads of theses organization.

The government and various social organizations in Manipur should come together and foster networking among all the likes of social Organizations. Study conducted within the aforesaid four FBO's whose approach to behavior change is through holistic counseling, it shows that behavior changes through these counseling has minimal cases of relapse than detoxification/ substitution model where the cases of relapse cases sky rocketed. Looking into the success and achievement of FBO's in the state of Manipur the state government through its various agencies can identify certain FBO's who are really doing well in their own part despite the size of the organization and fund their project so that the HIV sero-prevalence rate is reversed.

It can be concluded that on the part of the government efforts has been made and it is thus the collective responsibility of the government and various stake holders. It is difficult to come to any hard conclusions that politicians are really committed to HIV/AIDS mitigation in the state as stated earlier. Commitment is multidimensional and therefore, cannot be measured through a single quantitative indicator.

The respondents are happy with the services provided by the government and NGO's except for negligible number of respondents wanted government to provide drugs for opportunistic Infections and subsidized the rates of basic necessities for people living with HIV and AIDS.

APPENDICES

ANNEXURE 1

PROFILES OF IDUS, PLWHA AND BENEFICIARIES IN IMPHAL EAST AND WEST DISTRICT OF MANIPUR

Department of Social Work, Assam University, Silchar 788011

I am a PhD research scholar from Department of Social Work, Assam University Silchar. I am collecting information on services provided by the government and nongovernmental organisation from Beneficiaries/IDU's, PLWHA's point of view. In this regard I request your precious time in answering some of my question. The Information gathered during this process will be used solely for research purposes. I would be very thankful to you for your kind co-operation.

1. **Social background**

1.1	Respondent Number	:	....
1.2	Place of residence (Leikai)	:	....
1.3	Age	:	....
1.4	Sex	:	1) Male 2) Female 9) NA
1.5	Educational level	:	1) Primary 2) Secondary 3) Hr. Sec 4) Graduate 5) P.G 8) any other 9) NA
1.6	Religion	:	1) Hindu 2) Muslim 3) Christian 8) Any other 9) NA
1.7	Mother tongue	:	1) Manipuri 2) Hindi 3) Tribal Dialect 8) any other 9) NA
1.8	Are you employed/ working?	:	1) Yes 2) No 8) any other 9) NA

1.9 If yes, can you tell me the nature of employment? : 1) Government 2) NGO 3) Services 4) Business 5) Self employed 8) any other 9) NA

1.10 If not, can you cite some reason : 1) Personal/Family 2) Medical reason 3) Closure of establishment 8) any other 9) NA

1.10 a) Give details : ....

1.11 Marital status of the respondent : 1) Single 2) Engaged 3) Married 4) Divorced/separated 9) NA

1.12 What is the age of your spouse? : ....

1.13 What was your age when you got married?: ....

1.13 a) Actual number of years since married (Don't ask): ....

1.14 Are you staying/living together with your family? : 1) Yes 2) no 8) any other 9) NA

1.15 If living away, how long has it been now? : ....

1.15 a) Reason for living away : ....

1.16 Total monthly Income from all sources (Rupees): a) Respondent Rs................. only

b) Family/ Spouse Rs................. only

c) Total Income from a) &b) Rs................. only

1.17 What is the type of your family : 1) Nuclear 2) Joint family 3) Extended family 9) NA

1.18 How many members are there in your family? 1) 0 to 2 2) 3 to 4 3) 5 to 6 4) 7 to 8 5) 9 to 10 6) 11 and above 8) any other 9) NA

1.19 Are you financially dependent on your family? 1) Yes 2) no 8) any other 9) NA

1.20 How many members of your family are dependent on you? 1) 0 to 2 2) 3 to 4 3) 5 to 6 4) 7 to 8 5) 9 to 10 6) 11 and above 9) NA

1.21 If earning can you save some part of your earning : 1) yes 2) no 9) NA

2. **For Drug/Intoxication users and IDUs** (If the respondent is not an IDU leave the entire section)

2.1 Age at onset of oral drugs use : ....

2.2 Sources of drugs : 1) Pharmacy 2) Peer groups 3) Drug peddlers 8) any other 9) NA

2.2 a) Any other (Give Details) : ....

2.3 Types of drugs/Intoxication use

Types of Drugs Yes No Any other NA

a) Heroin

b) Diazepam

c)Spasmo proxyvon (SP)

d) Ganja/Marijuana

e) Nitrovite tablets

f) Cough syrups

g) Adhesive solution

h) Brown sugar

i) Tidigesic

j) Calmpose

k) Buprenorphine

l) Alcohol

	m) Any other		
2.4	If any other, give details	:	....
2.5	Frequency of drug/intoxication use daily	:	1) once 2) Twice 3) Thrice 4) four 5) five 6) More than five 8) any other 9) NA
2.6	Age at onset of Injecting drug use	:	....
2.7	Do you usually take drugs alone/in company		1) alone 2) In company of friends 8) any other 9) NA
2.8	Did you borrow/ lend/share injecting equipment during		
	a) The past	:	1) Yes 2) no 8) any other 9) NA
	b) Present	:	1) Yes 2) no 8) any other 9) NA
2.9	Did you ever give up using of drugs within this period	:	1) yes 2) no 9) NA
2.10	Periods of abstinence of drugs	:	1) 0 to 2 days 2) 2 to 4 days 3) 4 to 6 days 4) 6 days to 2 weeks 5) 2 to 4 weeks 6) 4 weeks to 6 weeks 7) 6 weeks or more 8) any other 9) NA
2.11	Have you ever been admitted to de-addiction/Rehabilitation centre (Within 1 year)	:	1) Yes 2) no 8) any other 9) NA
	If yes number of times	:	....
2.12	Who brought you/ referred you	:	1) Family 2) Relatives 3) Peer/ colleagues 8) any other 9) NA
2.13	What triggers you to relapse? (First three)	:	1) Peer pressure 2) anger 3) Loss of job 4) Depression 5) Family problem 8) any other 9) NA
2.13	a) what do you think is the main reason for your relapse (elaborate)	:	....

2.14	Do you know about any safer practices/injection		1) Yes 2) no 9) NA
2.15	If yes, what is it? (First Three)	:	1) Always using new equipment needles, syringes etc. 2) Before injecting removing any metals or rings which are close fitted 3) Shooting at arms or hand as the risk is low here because of good flow of blood 4) Alternating veins/ shooting area 5) Taking a deep breath and not to be in a hurry 6) If injecting alone to hit on the other hand 7) Taking help from others 8) any other 9) NA
2.16	Do you know of any substitution programme		1) Yes 2) no 9) NA
2.17	Did the NGO/Care centre provide any substitution for detoxification?	:	1) Yes 2) No 8) any other 9) NA
2.18	Have you ever taken drugs in overdose in anytime of your life?	:	1) Yes 2) no 9) NA
2.19	If yes, what measures did you take afterward	:	1) reduce my doses 2) seek advice from peer group 3) Consulted de-addiction centre/Doctors 8) any other 9) NA
2.20	what are the symptoms you experience when you cannot obtain drugs (Mark first three)	:	1) anxiety/craving 2) running nose/watering of eyes 3) Loose motion/diarrhea 4) slight fever 5) Muscle ache 6) sweating/ goose flesh 7) Nausea/vomiting 8) any other 9) NA

2.20a)	after obtaining drugs, elaborate on if you face any problem	:	....
2.21	How do you arrange funds for drugs	:	1) Daily wage 2) Selling household items/ goods 3) Pinching? 4) Asking from friends/ relatives/ family 8) any other 9) NA
2.22	What is your history of drug use	:	1) oral pills 2) Injecting 3) sniffing solution 8) any other 9) NA
2.23	If you have ever changed the way you consume/take drugs, can you give three reason?		1) To get more high/kick 2) To cut down cost 3) Peer pressure 4) to experience new way of taking drugs 8) Any other 9) NA
2.24	How do you clean up your injecting equipment?	:	1) Cleaning with disinfectant 2) Cleaning with water 3) Boiling/ Sterilization 4) Using new equipment 8) any other 9) NA
2.25	How do you dispose off your injecting equipment?	:	1) Disposing at the Nullah 2) Disposing at the river 3) Throwing at the waste bin 4) Burning the needle 8) any other 9) NA
3.	**Illness and Medical History**		
3.1	Can I ask you few questions on your medical history,		
	Have you ever had fever/ cough during the past six months?	:	1) Yes 2) no 8) any other 9) NA
3.2	How long does it last?	:	1) 0 to 2 days 2) 2 to 4 days 3) 4 days to 1 week 4) 1 week to 2 weeks 5) More than 2 weeks 8) any other 9) NA
3.3	Do you meet any Doctor/Medical professional?	:	1) Yes 2) No 9) NA

3.4	If yes, please specify?	:	1) Registered Medical practitioner 2) Private Medical practitioner 3) Self medication 7) Use of home remedy 8) any other 9) NA
3.5	Looking into the last three years of your life, have you ever suffered from an illness which require investigations of the following: Investigations	:	Yes No Any other NA Blood investigation (Don't ask. Typhoid, Malaria, TB, Hepatitis, Liver disease, STI, HIV) Liver disease, STI, HIV)X Rays/Ultra sound Other diagnostic investigation Any other
3.6	If yes to any one above, did this require hospitalization	:	1) Yes 2) No 8) any other 9) NA
3.7	If yes did you undergo any surgery/ blood transfusion (if yes go to Q no. 4.17)	:	1) Yes 2) No 8) any other 9) NA
4.	**HIV/STI Knowledge, risk perception and HIV test uptake**		
4.1	As we all know what TB is, I hope you are aware of it	:	1) Yes 2) No 8) any other 9) NA
4.2	Have you ever had a history of TB in your life	:	1) Yes 2) No 8) any other 9) NA
4.3	Have you heard about Hepatitis?	:	1) Yes 2) No 8) any other 9) NA
4.4	If yes, what is Hepatitis?	:	1) A virus which cause inflammation of the liver 2) Have little knowledge about it 3) Have no idea 8) any other 9) NA

4.5	What are the different types of Hepatitis	:	1) Hepatitis A 2) Hepatitis B 3) Hepatitis C 4) Hepatitis D 5) Hepatitis E 6) Hepatitis G 7) all the above 8) any other 9) NA
4.6	What are the symptoms of Hepatitis C?	:	1) Headache 2) Fever 3) Chills 4) General weakness 5) Jaundice 6) all the above 7) have no Idea 9) NA
4.7	How can it be transmitted from one person to another?	:	1) Contaminated blood transfusion 2) Sexual contacts 3) Using of infected needles/syringes 7) have no idea 8) any other 9) NA
4.8	Have you heard about STI/STD	:	1) Yes 2) no 8) any other 9) NA
4.9	How does it spread from one person to another?	:	1) Sexual contact 2) have no idea 8) any other 9) NA
4.10	What are the different types of STI/STD? (First three)	:	1) Syphilis 2) Gonorrhea 3) Chlamydia 4) Chancroid 5) Trichomoniosis 6) Herpes simplex virus 7) Genital ulcer 8) any other 9) NA
4.11	What are the symptoms of STI/STD (first three)	:	1) Vaginal discharge2) Inguinal bubo/ inflammation of the groin 3) Pelvic inflammatory 4) genital ulcers/ Herpes 5) Pain on passing urine/discharge of puss 6) pain/blisters in the genital region 7) Formation of lesion 8) any other 9) NA
4.12	How do you acquire information on STI	:	1) From parents and relative 2) From friends 3) from NGO 4) Pamphlets/leaflets 5) TV/ Radio 6) school/college 7) Advertisement and hoardings 8) Hospital 9) NA
4.13	As we all know about HIV/AIDS, did you?	:	1) Yes 2) no 8) any other 9) NA

4.14	If yes, where from did you get to know about it?		1) From parents and relative 2) From friends 3) from NGO 4) Pamphlets/leaflets 5) TV/ Radio 6) school/college 7) advertisement and hoardings 8) Any other 9) NA
4.15	What are the different modes of HIV transmission?	:	1) Unprotected Sexual intercourse 2) Infected needles and syringes 3) Infected blood transfusion 4) From infected mother to child 7) all the above 8) any other 9) NA
4.16	How can one prevent oneself from HIV/STI	:	1) abstinence from sex 2) being faithful to sexual partners 3) using of condoms while having sexual intercourse 4) Receiving blood from authorized blood banks 5) Regular check up for STI/ STD 6) All the above 8) any other 9) NA
4.17	If surgery/ blood transfusion were done could you tell me the result of blood examination, was HIV+?	:	1) Yes 2) no 8) any other 9) NA
4.18	What is ART	:	1) It is Anti Retro Viral Therapy 2) It is a drugs to slow down the spread of HIV virus 7) All the above 8) Any other 9) NA
4.19	Name any Govt. ART centers in Imphal?	:	1) RIMS Hospital 2) J.N Hospital 3) Both 1 & 2 4) No Idea 8) Any other 9) NA
4.20	Are you in contact / in touch with any NGO's or GO's	:	1) yes 2) no 8) any other 9) NA
4.21	If yes, what are the services you received from (first three)		
4.21a)	Government	:	1) Counseling 2) Referral services 3) Clinical test 4) Treatment & prevention services 8) any other 9) NA

4.21b) Non-Government Organisation : 1) Counseling 2) Referral services 3) Clinical test 4) Treatment & prevention services 5) Detoxification for drugs 6) Needle and syringe exchange program 7) all of the above 8) any other 9) NA

4.22 Do you feel the services you received were adequate to meet your needs?

4.22a) Government : 1) Yes 2) no 9) NA

4.22b) Non-Governmental organisation : 1) Yes 2) no 9) NA

4.23 If not give reason (specify Government and Non Government separately) ....

5. **Sexual History**

5.1 Usually young boys and girls have relationship before marriage, do you experience it?

1) Yes 2) no 8) any other 9) NA

5.2 At what age did you experience sexual initiation : ....

5.3 How often do you use condom during your sexual activity with your partner (During last year)

: 1) Every time 2) quite often 3) sometimes when it is available 8) any other 9) NA

5.3a) If using give reason : 1) to avoid pregnancy2) Protect one from STD/STI, HIV/AIDS 3) Both 1 and 2 8) Any other 9) NA

5.3 b) If not using give reason : 1) It reduce sexual pleasure 2) Non availability 8) any other 9) NA

5.4 Do you visit commercial sex workers?

5.5a) Past : 1) Yes 2) no 9) NA

5.5b) Present : 1) Yes 2) no 9) NA

5.5 If yes, how often do you visit in a month? : 1) Once 2) twice 3) thrice 4) four 5) More than four times 8) any other 9) NA

5.6 How often do you use condom during such encounters? : 1) every time 2) quite often 3) sometimes when it is available 8) Any other 9) NA

5.6a) If yes give reason : 1) to avoid pregnancy 2) Protect one from STD/STI, HIV/AIDS 3) Both 1 and 2 8) Any other 9) NA

5.6b) If not give reason : 1) It reduce sexual pleasure 2) Non availability 8) any other 9) NA

5.7 Do you have sexual encounter with other IDUs/ MSM : 1) Yes 2) No 8) any other 9) NA

5.8 If yes, how often do you have? : 1) Once 2) twice 3) thrice 4) four 5) More than four times 8) Any other 9) NA

5.9 Do you use condom in such activity : 1) Yes 2) no 8) any other 9) NA

5.10 How often do you use condom during : 1) every time 2) quite often 3) Sometimes when it is available

such encounters : 8) any other 9) NA

5.10a) If yes give reason : 1) to avoid pregnancy 2) Protect one from STD/STI, HIV/AIDS 3) Both 1 and 2 8) Any other 9) NA

5.10b) If not give reason : 1) It reduce sexual pleasure 2) Non availability 8) any other 9) NA

6. Imprisonment and drug use in jail (If the respondent is not an IDU leave the entire section)

6.1 Have you ever been caught by the police for your drug use? 1) Yes 2) No 8) any other 9) NA

6.2 Have you ever been imprisoned for your drug use or your HIV status? 1) Yes 2) No 8) any other 9) NA

6.3 Have you ever been imprisoned for your drug use or your HIV status? 1) Yes 2) No 8) any other 9) NA

6.4 Did you ever use drugs inside the jail premises? 1) Yes 2) No 8) any other 9) NA

6.5 Would you like to share the sources of your drugs? 1) Yes 2) No 8) any other 9) NA

6.6 Where did you get those drugs? 1) From peer and colleagues 2) From the jail staff 3) Family/ relatives 8) any other 9) NA

6.7 What are the sources of funds 1) From peer and colleagues 2) From the jail staff? 3) Family/ relatives 8) any other 9) NA

6.8 Do you feel the need to introduce awareness program inside the jail premises 1) Yes 2) No 8) any other 9) NA

6.9 If yes, on which component according to you the government/NGO should stressed their awareness program inside the jail premises (first Three) 1) Legal rights 2) IEC 3) Treatment 4) Care /support 5) After care 8) any other 9) NA

Note: not to be asked (Probe deep) outstanding charges, ever been banned by any social organization

7. Benefits received from Government or non governmental organisation

7.1 Did you get supply of needles and syringes regularly from the?

7.1a) Government : 1) Yes 2) No 8) any other 9) NA

7.1b) NGO : 1) Yes 2) No 8) any other 9) NA

7.2 Have you ever been treated/admitted for treatment of TB /HIV in Hospital 1) Yes 2) No 8) any other 9) NA

7.2a) if yes give details ....

7.3 Did you get access to ART treatment in?

7.3a) Government hospital : 1) Yes 2) No 8) any other 9) NA

7.3b) NGO : 1) Yes 2) No 8) any other 9) NA

7.3c) Give details about your experience (Availability of drugs, Doctors, counseling services and any discrimination)

....

7.4 Did you ever face any discrimination in family/ society/ community, any set up? (Elaborate) ....

7.5 Are you satisfied with the level of government/NGO/FBO/CBO interventions? : 1) Yes 2) No 8) any other 9) NA

7.6 If not satisfied which component should the government/NGO/FBO/CBO give priority? (First three) : 1) Legal rights 2) IEC 3) Treatment 4) Care /support 5) Hospice care 6) Mobile STI clinic, ICTC 7) Hospice 8) Needles/Syringes exchange 9) NA

8. **Understanding about the government policies and programmes on HIV and AIDS**

8.1 Do you know NACP III : 1) Yes 2) No 8) any other 9) NA

8.2 Rate your level of understanding of the various components of NACP III Programmes : Very good Good Fair Any other NA

Prevention (T.I, STI Care, ICTC, Blood Safety, IEC, Condom promotion)

Care (Treatment of O.I, Provision of free DOT treatments, PEP, ART)

Collaboration (GIPA, Inter sectoral collaboration, Involvement of ministries, workplace intervention etc.)

Capacity building (Programme management, AIDS vaccine initiative, M&E etc.)

9. **General observation of the respondent by the scholar**

Thank you once again

ANNEXURE 2

INTERVIEW SCHEDULE FOR FUNCTIONARIES

Department of Social Work , Assam University, Silchar 788011

I am a PhD research scholar from Department of Social Work, Assam University Silchar. I am collecting information on services provided by the government and non governmental organisation from Beneficiaries/IDU's, PLWHA's, Political leaders, Administrative heads, F.B.O's point of view. In this regard I request your precious time in answering some of my question. The Information gathered during this process will be used solely for research purposes. I would be very thankful to you for your kind co-operation.

1. **Profile of the functionary**

a) Name of the respondent

b) Age

c) Sex

d) Marital status

e) Religion

f) Educational Qualification

g) Professional Qualification

h) Number of years in service (Total)

i) Number of years in service in this organisation

j) Job Description (Nature of task)

k) Income

i) Salary :....................

ii) From other sources (if any) :....................

iii) Total....................

2. Name of the organisation : ....
3. Objectives of the organisation : ....
4. Number of employees (i) permanent : ....
   (ii) Temporary : ....
   (iii) Voluntary : ....
   (iv) Male and female employment ratio : ....
5. When did your organisation start HIV/AIDS intervention programme
6. Does your organisation have HIV/AIDS prevention programmes of the following? (Multiple response permissible)
   HIV/AIDS Prevention education in schools/colleges and institutions : 1) Yes 2) No 9) NA
   HIV/AIDS awareness programmes in the communities : 1) Yes 2) No 9) NA
   Developing and disseminating IEC material : 1) Yes 2) No 9) NA
   Provision of counselling services ; 1) Yes 2) No 9) NA
   Peer education : 1) Yes 2) No 9) NA
   Drama/ Leella or any other folk media : 1) Yes 2) No 9) NA
   Condom promotion/distribution : 1) Yes 2) No 9) NA
7. According to your experience, what do you think is the most effective of all prevention programmes listed above?
   ....

8. What are the challenges you faced in implementing prevention programmes

....

....

Consider if your organisation have the following care and support services

General health care to PLWHA	:	1) Yes	2) No	9) NA
STI treatment /management	:	1) Yes	2) No	9) NA
TB-HIV co-infection management	:	1) Yes	2) No	9) NA
Palliative (reducing the severity of disease symptom) care	:	1) Yes	2) No	9) NA
Referral services	:	1) Yes	2) No	9) NA
Paediatric (infant and child care) aids treatment	:	1) Yes	2) No	9) NA
Home based care	:	1) Yes	2) No	9) NA
Collaboration with other NGO's and care centre	:	1) Yes	2) No	9) NA
Nutritional support	:	1) Yes	2) No	9) NA

9. What are the challenges you faced while providing care and support services:

....

....

Consider if you provide the following services to your clients

Financial support	:	1) Yes	2) No	9) NA
Financial support for ration/clothes etc	:	1) Yes	2) No	9) NA
Vocational training to PLWHA	:	1) Yes	2) No	9) NA
Assistance in job Placement	:	1) Yes	2) No	9) NA

Self help group formation : 1) Yes 2) No 9) NA

Educational support for children affected/infected by HIV/AIDS : 1)Yes 2)No 9) NA

Facilitation of PLWHA network ; 1) Yes 2) No 9) NA

10. Comment on the above services (response and its effectiveness) : ....

Do you have any of these programme management services:

Information sharing through publication of journals, newsletter etc : 1) Yes 2) No9) NA

Participate in planning process of MACS : 1) Yes 2) No 9) NA

Capacity building programme for health care workers and community leaders

: 1)Yes 2) No 9) NA

Provide the services of resource persons : 1) Yes 2) No 9) NA

Clinical research : 1) Yes 2) No 9) NA

Social research : 1) Yes 2) No 9) NA

11. What are the challenges and difficulties you faced in management of the above services : ....

In the state of Manipur what would be your recommendation for an effective strategy for the prevention of HIV/AIDS:

....

12. The area you work in is a sensitive one, kindly discuss the skills and competencies that make you an effective worker with the AIDS afflicted people:........ ....

Do you have to take precautionary measures: If yes, please elaborate? : ....

13. No doubt, you must be undergoing Stress (Job related) how do you cope up with it? :..................................

14. Can you suggest the diverse roles and responsibilities of a professional social workers in the context of HIV/AIDS (Ask if Applicable

....

15. Going to some personal questions, can you rate the satisfaction level of your job : 1. Not so satisfied
2) Moderately satisfied
3) Satisfied
4) highly satisfied
8) Any other
9) NA

16. If not satisfied please give reason : ....

Thank you once again

ANNEXURE 3

INTERVIEW GUIDE FOR POLITICIANS

Department Of Social Work , Assam University, Silchar 788011

I am a PhD research scholar from Department of Social Work, Assam University Silchar. I am collecting information on services provided by the governmental and non governmental organisation from Beneficiaries/IDU's, PLWHA's, Political leaders, Administrative heads, and representatives of F.B.O's. In this regard I request your precious time in answering some of my questions. The Information gathered during this process will be used solely for research purposes. I would be very thankful to you for your kind co-operation.

Name of the respondent (*not to be asked)*

Name of the political Party you belong to (*not to be asked)*

1. Sir/Madam you must be familiar with the gravity of HIV/AIDS. Do you think AIDS is a political issue? If yes/no why
2. Kindly share with me whether you have been involved in any forum or in any programme of HIV/AIDS awareness and prevention (give detail)
3. Does affiliation to a particular party affect your stand with respect to social issues such as HIV/AIDS? Yes/no please elaborate
4. Have you been approached by the media to talk about the issue of HIV/AIDS

5. Are you wiling to espouse and stand for the cause of HIV/ AIDS mitigation in your constituency? Intended plan of action. If not kindly give reason
6. Are you satisfied with the manner of surveillance and reporting of HIV/AIDS in our state? Yes/no please elaborate
7. According to you what are the priority issues pertaining to HIV/AIDS (stigma, prevention and treatment, targeted intervention for specific groups)
8. Please elaborate on the priority of the assembly budget allocation for HIV/AIDS
9. Can you give an estimate of your local area development fund being utilised for the causes of HIV/AIDS
10. Has there been any special session in the state assembly for HIV/AIDS (resolution passed if any)
11. Sir/Madam please comment on the funding patterns (*in the context of organisations working on HIV/AIDS, nature, type, utilization etc e.g project orchid)*
    a) Government funding
    b) Foreign funding
    c) Fund raising by NPO
12. Manipur stands out to be a state which has a specific policy on HIV/AIDS since 1996, kindly comment on the direction it has given to AIDS programming in your state (Best practices)
13. Sir/Madam are you aware of any forum at the national level (convenor)

Sir/Madam let me have your views on the legislative procedures available for AIDS

14. Do you think that the existing legislative procedure allows for a well grounded discussion on HIV/AIDS yes/no? In your experience what has been the best time to raise questions on this issue (0 hour, Q hour, call attention motion hour etc)

15. I would like to ask you your personal contribution in terms of starred and unstarred questions raised in the legislative proceedings regarding the issue of HIV/AIDS
16. Please comment on the nature and frequency of constituency specific issues and client specific questions in legislative proceedings if any...vis a vis HIV/AIDS
17. Please comment on the manifesto of all major national and state political outfit vis a vis health (HIV/AIDS)
18. What is the mission, vision and objectives of Manipur legislative forum on HIV/AIDS
19. What do you think are the major areas we have to work on for best implementation of our AIDS control policy in the state of Manipur?
20. What is the role and contribution of Manipur legislative forum on HIV/AIDS? What more roles can it play? (Conference, training, stigma, Discrimination etc)
21. Has the state government involved different department/ ministries to combat the problems of HIV/AIDS? If yes/ no please elaborate
22. I would like to have your comment on the infrastructural, institutional, manpower and service availability in our state particularly in the public health care sector for PLWHA (sufficient no. of hospital Beds, availability of trained medical professionals, requisite no. of ICTC, ART Centre, sufficient supply of screened blood etc)
23. Sir/Madam please comment on the nature of intervention at schools and university by the state in terms of HIV/AIDS mitigation (University
24. Does the government have any plan to draft a state law to protect the rights of PLWHA or if there is any future plan, please comment on it
25. Do you think that there has been a significant political will in your state to tackle the problem of HIV/AIDS? Please support your answer with specific instances.

Thank you once again

ANNEXURE 4

INTERVIEW GUIDE FOR FAITH BASED ORGANISATION

Department of Social Work, Assam University, Silchar 788011

I am a PhD research scholar from Department of Social Work, Assam University Silchar. I am collecting information on services provided by the government and non governmental organisation from Beneficiaries/IDU's, PLWHA's, Political leaders, Administrative heads, F.B.O's point of view. In this regard I request your precious time in answering some of my question. The Information gathered during this process will be used solely for research purposes. I would be very thankful to you for your kind co-operation

Background Information

1. Name of the respondent (details- Sex, Age, Educational Qualification, years of service in the organisation)
2. Name of the organisation
3. How long has it been functioning
4. What is your organisation religious affiliation
5. Organisational hierarchy
6. Number of employees (i) permanent

    (ii) Temporary

    (iii) Voluntary

    (iv) Male and female employment ratio

7. Main objectives of the organisation

Start Conversation

8. How is your organisation registered (Societies registration Act, Companies Act etc)
9. Details of staff educational qualification

Number of staff with post Graduate Degree	....
Number of staff with Graduate Degree	....
Number of staff studying up to 12 Std.	....
Number of staff studying up to 10 Std	....
Number of staff under 10 Std	....

10. Recruitment - (Advertisement to Interview and giving offer letter e.g. Tel. int. preliminary test, main test, interview. Simple, self referral & others)

Induction process of the staff (Training)

11. Does educational qualification have anything to do in the selection process (if yes give examples)
12. Is faith affiliation of the applicant to the job in your organisation an important criteria in the selection process
13. Are there any staff who follows other faith

Taking our conversation forward, let us talk about your organisations, HIV/AIDS intervention programme

14. (Probe deep) let us discuss about your organisation projects, programme, Target groups, funding patterns and collaboration.

Last 3 Years Project	Program-mes	Target Groups PLWHA/ HRG'S	Funding Agencies NGO'S	Collaboration Govt/

15. What initiated your organisation into taking up HIV/AIDS intervention programme

16. In your opinion, employees working in your organisation on HIV/AIDS, STI etc are well aware of the issues and special needs of the beneficiaries of your programmes

17. If some employees are not and needs a training , what remedial measures did you take in this regard (counselling, sharing problems etc

18. Looking back up to the last 3 years, have you or other employees attended any training programme on HIV/AIDS

19. If possible would you like to share with me if any HIV+ person employed in your organisation (HOLD)

20. What does your programme on HIV/AIDS focus on (Give details)

    a) BCC

    b) Condom Promotion {View, Promotion/Distribution-(Free, Social Marketing)}

    c) STI Management

    d) I.E.C (Pamphlets, Posture, Puppet Shows, Folk Media etc)

    e) Counselling (Psychological aspect)

21. Where do you usually refer your clients to (Home based care, drop in centre, Hospital etc)

22. Do you have a follow up services for your clients after referring them to the ICTC

23. If not referred, what have been the steps your organisation has initiated (Most of the clients) to cope with their illness (HIV/AIDS)

    (F.B Counselling, Access to Medicines and Treatment, home visits/ home based care, Hospice care, Employment/ Financial Support etc)

24. What policy on HIV prevention would you like to see, other faith organisations to encourage (Optional)
25. What could be done in your opinion to share accountability for HIV prevention across faith organisations in national setting
26. What Monitoring and evaluation techniques did your organisation adopt for your programme for its effectiveness (Give details)
27. Have you ever been a member or a part of a consultation group in state, national and international level
28. If yes, what were the issues focussed upon and what was your role
29. Are you aware of the NACP III
30. If yes would you like to share/comment upon NACP III on prevention, Care, Support and Treatment
31. At large, how are FBO'S perceived to have contributed to the formation of HIV/AIDS policy in Manipur
32. Can you give an example on how FBO made a difference in the fight against HIV/AIDS anywhere on the globe
33. In the state of Manipur what would be your recommendation for an effective strategy for the prevention of HIV/AIDS
34. What have been the major challenges/obstacles faced by you in your programme on HIV/AIDS
35. In your opinion, Are F.B.O'S adequately funded to provide services to PLWHA, the vulnerable and the high risk groups
36. What in your opinion would bring about effective/optimum utilisation of the funds/other resources of an F.B.O'S to communities providing support to P.L.W.H.A, the vulnerable and H.R.G'S
37. Are there any biases in funding which tend to support larger, well established F.B.O'S

Thank you once again

ANNEXURE 5

INTERVIEW GUIDE FOR SOCIAL AND CULTURAL ORGANISATION

Department of Social Work, Assam University, Silchar 788011

I am a PhD research scholar from Department of Social Work, Assam University Silchar. I am collecting information on services provided by the governmental and non governmental organisation from Beneficiaries/IDU's, PLWHA's, Political leaders, Administrative heads, Functionaries, F.B.O's, Notable person's/ civil societies in the field of HIV/AIDS point of view. In this regard I request your precious time in answering some of my questions. The information gathered during this process will be used solely for research purposes.

I would be very thankful to you for your kind co-operation.

Name of the respondent (*optional*) ....

1. Position in the organisation
2. History of the organisation *(when did you start working for the cause of HIV/AIDS patient? What are your target groups)*
3. Objectives of the organisation
4. In the past five years what major issues have been addressed by your organisation, so as to bring about change in the society *(give examples of successful programme)*
5. How do you mobilize community participation in the programme of HIV/AIDS addressed by your organisation? *(give details and example of advocacy)*
6. As we know drug use is very much related to the spread of HIV/AIDS, what are the initiatives that your organisation

has taken up to mitigate the problem of HIV/AIDS

7. With respect to NSEP (*needle and syringe exchange programme)* what is your strategy on this (*details)*
8. Going into details, what has been the nature of work for the control of drug abuse by your organisation
9. Do you have any difficulties in executing your objectives (reason)
10. Kindly elaborate on the nature of fund raising activities that support your programmes

for meira paibi's and AMADA

11.Drawing your attention towards the problems of HIV/AIDS, please give me more information

a) Are you satisfied the way government is working especially in the field of HIV/AIDS Mitigation

b) Did the government provide enough facilities in the hospital (*Blood bank/Units, Beds, Medicine, Nutrition's etc*)

c) Did the government give enough provisions for PLWHA, Children and the orphan

d) MACS is the Nodal agency for prevention, care & support of HIV/AIDS. Do they work enough to meet the aspirations of the local people?

e) Do we have requisite number of ICTC's to cater to the needs of the people

12. Does your organisation have any collaboration with other organisations such as F.B.Os. C.B.O's, NGO's etc
13. What role did your organisation play in removing stigma and discrimination attached with PLWHA?
14. Future plans of the organisation (*Tie up with NGO's and other course of action in the prevention of HIV/AIDS)*
15. What are the suggestion you would like to make, if any for the effective containment of HIV/AIDS infection (socio-economic, empowerment)

Thank you once again

for Meira Paibis and AMADA

ANNEXURE 6

INTERVIEW GUIDE FOR SACS, ICMR AND NOTABLE PERSONS IN THE FIELD OF HIV/AIDS

Department of Social Work, Assam University, Silchar 788011

I am a PhD research scholar from Department of Social Work, Assam University Silchar. I am collecting information on services provided by the governmental and non governmental organisation from Beneficiaries/IDU's, PLWHA's, Political leaders, Administrative heads, Functionaries, F.B.O's, Notable person's in the field of HIV/AIDS point of view. In this regard I request your precious time in answering some of my questions. The information gathered during this process will be used solely for research purposes. I would be very thankful to you for your kind co-operation.

Name of the respondent: ....

Name of the organisation: ....

1. As we well know that Manipur is proud to have its own policy on AIDS since 1996
   a) What have been the major initiatives at the state level
   b) What direction has this policy given to AIDS prevention and control?
   c) What are the major gaps in our policy?(*Your suggestion for filling this)*
2. By and large HIV testing is on a voluntary basis, but do

we have mandatory testing requirement in any situation such as (employment, marriage, travel, or access to health care services)

3. No doubt people's participation is important in making any programme successful, has there been so with the AIDS programme(give example)
4. Do you think we have sufficient services in the following areas in our state
   a. Condom availability (Social Marketing, Vending machine etc)
   b. STI diagnosis and treatment facilities (Mobile clinics)
   c. ICTC'S (counselling services, maintaining confidentiality)
   d. IEC materials on HIV prevention
   e. Sufficient hospital beds/ hospice care for the HIV/AIDS infected in our state
5. Manipur AIDS policy in the context of drug use focuses on harm minimization, what major activities are carried out to achieve this? (Needle Exchange, Substitution treatment, peer education, condom promotion etc)
6. As you know that AIDS is no more restricted to drug users, it has been reported extensively in the general population. What specific programme exist for the general population (*women and children, truckers, migrant population etc*)
7. No doubt a large number of programmes are going on in our state, can you please comment on the effectiveness of the RIAC (*positive and negative aspect)*
8. a) Can you please comment on the major achievement in our state in the last five years in the control of HIV/AIDS

   b) What have been some of our major target (goals) to combat the epidemic and how well have they been achieved

c) If these targets have not been achieved (ART centres, Hospice care, de-addiction centres, no. of hospital beds, social marketing of condoms) what have been the major reason (financial support, political commitment, availability of manpower etc)

9. Do you think the programme on HIV/AIDS in the state of Manipur are supported with sufficient funds/and manpower

   a) Government funding

   b) Foreign funding

   c) Fund raising by NPO etc.

10 a) Have you come across any instance of stigma and discrimination in the last one year for HIV infected person, give details

   b) What are your suggestions to address the problem of stigma and discrimination *(Law, work place policy etc?)*

11. What is the status of sentinel and behavioural surveillance of HIV/AIDS in our state? What remedial measures would you like to suggest if any

12. Inherent to successful programming in the techniques of monitoring and evaluation, kindly comment in the context of your organisation (ask if applicable)

13. What is your opinion on the nature of partnerships between different torch bearers in the control of HIV/AIDS (NGO'S, FBO'S, Civil Society Organisations, Private organisations- *best example?*)

14. Please comment on the nature of training of the human resources for HIV/AIDS programme in the state; give details (*Doctor's, Nurses, Teachers, functionaries, counsellors etc*)

15. What in your opinion is the benefit of using more behavioural change approach and having more programs on counselling, developing peer support groups etc? Your suggestion please

16. What is your opinion on greater investment in training and development of manpower to carry out the HIV/AIDS programme?
17. Apart from above discussion, kindly comment on the policy, program and strategy of HIV/AIDS in the state of Manipur

Thank you once again

ANNEXURE 7

INTERVIEW GUIDE FOR ADMINISTRATIVE HEADS

Department of Social Work, Assam University, Silchar 788011

I am a PhD research scholar from Department of Social Work, Assam University Silchar. I am collecting information on services provided by the government and non governmental organisation from Beneficiaries/IDU's, PLWHA's, Political leaders, Administrative heads, Functionaries, F.B.O's, Notable person's in the field of HIV/AIDS point of view. In this regard I request your precious time in answering some of my question. The Information gathered during this process will be used solely for research purposes. I would be very thankful to you for your kind co-operation.

1. Name of the respondent (details- Sex, Age, Educational Qualification, years of service in the organisation)
2. Name of the organisation
3. How long has it been functioning
4. Objectives of the organisation
5. Number of employees
   (i) permanent
   (ii) Temporary
   (iii) Voluntary
   (iv) Male and female employment ratio

6. Details of staff educational qualification
7. Recruitment- (Advertisement to Interview and giving offer letter eg. Tel. int. preliminary test, main test, interview)

    a) Induction process of the staff (Training)

8. Does educational qualification have anything to do in the selection process

    Taking our conversation forward, let us talk about your organisations, HIV/AIDS intervention programme

9. (Probe deep) let us discuss about your organisation projects, programme, Target groups, funding patterns and collaboration.

Last 3 Years Project	Program-mes	Target Groups PLWHA/ HRG'S	Funding Agencies NGO'S	Collaboration Govt/

POLICIES

10. As we well know that Manipur is proud to have its own policy on AIDS since 1996

    a) What direction has this policy given to AIDS prevention and control?

    b) What are the major gaps in our policy?

    Your suggestion for filling this

11. a) Can you please comment on the major achievement in our state in the last five years in the control of HIV/AIDS

    b) Shortfall of target has been because of (financial support, political commitment, availability of manpower etc)

12. What is your opinion in partnership between different torch bearers in the control of HIV/AIDS (NGO'S, FBO'S, Civil Society Organisations, Private organisations- best example)

PROGRAMMES

13. No doubt a large number of programmes are going on in our state, can you please comment on the effectiveness of the RIAC (Positive and Negative aspect)
14. As you know that AIDS is no more restricted to drug users, it has been reported extensively in the general population. What specific programme exist for women and children (PMTCT, Importance of women empowerment)
15. No doubt people's participation is important in making any programme successful, has there been so with the AIDS programme
16. What is the status of sentinel and behavioural surveillance of HIV/AIDS in our state? What remedial measures would you like to suggest if any
17. By and large HIV testing is a voluntary basis, but do we have mandatory testing requirement in any situation such as (employment, marriage, travel, or access to health care services
18. Have you come across any instance of stigma and discrimination in the last one year for HIV infected person, give details
19. What are your suggestions to address the problem of stigma and discrimination (Law, work place policy etc)
20. Manipur AIDS policy focus on harm minimization, what major activities are carried out to achieve this? (Needle Exchange, Substitution treatment, peer education, condom promotion etc)
21. Please comment on the nature of training of the human resources in the state, give details (Doctor's, Teachers, functionaries, counsellors etc)

22. Do you think we have sufficient services in the following areas in our state

    a) Condom availability (Social Marketing, Vending machine etc)

    b) STI diagnosis and treatment facilities (Mobile clinics)

    c) ICTC'S (counselling services, maintaining confidentiality)

    d) IEC materials on HIV prevention

23. Do you think that funding from international organisation/ corporate gives greater flexibility and better results

24. What alternative sources of fund raising have been successfully used by your organisation which has come to your notice (Ask if applicable)

25. Inherent to successful programming in the techniques of monitoring and evaluation , kindly comment in the context of your organisation (ask if applicable)

STRATEGIES

26. The strategy of HIV prevention in Manipur has been harm minimization in the context of IDU'S, do you think our programme has been able to meet its target (reason yes or no)

27. Could we have followed a more behavioural change approach and had wider programs such as counselling, developing peer support groups etc. your suggestion please

28. Do you think we would have achieved better results with greater investment in training and developing manpower to carry out the programme? Your suggestion please.

Sir/Madam thank you very much for your invaluable information, I hope and pray that this would help org/govt in formulating or in suggesting policy for a better life especially for PLWHA

Thank you once again

Bibliography

1. Agarwal AK, Singh GB, Khondon KC, Singh ND, Singh T, Jana S (1999). "*The prevalence of HIV in female sex workers in Manipur, India.*" The Journal of Communicable Diseases, Vol. 31, No. 1, pp. 23-8
2. Ahmed SI, (8-12 Nov. 1992, 1997) "*Truck Drivers as a vulnerable group in the North East India*". Abstract book of the 2nd International Congress on AIDS in ASIA and the pacific Ashok Hotel, New Delhi. (8-12 Nov. 1992, 1997)
3. Ahuja, R (2003) *Research Methods*. Rawat Publications, New Delhi
4. Archbishop Emeritus Desmond Tutu. *Video address to breaking the silence. Religious Health Organisations speak out on HIV and AIDS symposium, South Africa. July 2000*
5. Arjun BY, Unnikrishnan B, Ramapuram JT, Thapar R, Mithra P, Kumar N, Madi D, Kulkarni V, Holla R, Darshan B (2015) "*Factors Influencing Quality of Life among People Living with HIV in Coastal South India*". Journal of International Association Providers of AIDS Care. 2015 Aug 6.
6. Arndt, C and Lewis, J D (2001): "*The HIV/AIDS Pandemic in South Africa : Sectoral Impacts and Unemployment*", Journal of International Development, 13, 427-449, (2001)

7. Aruldas V., S. Abraham, T. Ninan., (2008) "Ideology matters: a framework for church policy on HIV/AIDS AIDS 2008" *XVII International AIDS Conference Abstracts book 2 pp 567 • 3-8 August 2008, Mexico City*
8. Aruldas V., S. Abraham, T. Ninan., (2008) Ideology matters: a framework for church policy on HIV and AIDS. *AIDS 2008 XVII International AIDS Conference Abstracts book 2 pp 567 • 3-8 August 2008, Mexico City*
9. Asian Harm Reduction Network (AHRN, 2001) "*HIV among Drug Injectors: The Hidden Epidemic in South East and East Asia*" (http:/www.ahrn.net/regional/overview.html) Accessed on 4/9/2014
10. Asian Harm Reduction Network (AHRN, 2001) "*HIV among Drug Injectors: The Hidden Epidemic in South East and East Asia*" (http:/www.ahrn.net/regional/overview.html) Accessed on 4/9/2014
11. Assessment of client satisfaction on capacity building and grant-making initiatives: the case of AMREF Maanisha Project in Kenya *AIDS 2008 XVII International AIDS Conference Abstracts book 2 pp 294 • 3-8 August 2008, Mexico City*
12. Athena P Kourtis MD, Francis K Lee PhD, Prof Elaine J Abrams MD, Denise J Jamieson MD, Marc Bulterys MD Nov (2006): "*Mother-to-child transmission of HIV-1: timing and implications for prevention*". The Lancet Infectious Diseases, Vol. 6 No. 11 pp 726-732
13. *Australia NSW HIV Strategy 2012–2015 A NEW ERA © NSW Ministry of Health 2012 SHPN 120419 ISBN 978-1-74187-853-0*
14. Bansal RK, Besarati Nia A., (1998) *"Truck crew and risk of contraction of STDS, including HIV: encouraging the use of condoms by the method of applying theories"*. Indian Journal of Medical Science. 1998 Jun; 52(6):253-64.
15. Barnett, T. School of Development Studies, University of East Anglia, Norwich NR4 7TJ, UK And Alan Whiteside "*Health Economics and HIV/AIDS*" Research Division,

University of Natal Durban 4041, South Africa Case Studies and a Conceptual Framework

16. Beyrer C, Razak MH, Lisam K, Chen J, Lui W, Yu XF (2000). *"Overland heroin trafficking routes and HIV-1 spread in south and south-east Asia."* AIDS, Vol. 14, No. 1, pp. 75-83
17. Beyrer, S., M. H. Razak, et al. (2000). *"Overland heroin trafficking routes and HIV-1 spread in south and south-east Asia."* AIDS, Vol. 14, No. 1, pp. 75-83.
18. Bhagat O.,(2003) *"Patterns of Ethnic Conflict in the North-East"* Economic and Political Weekly, May 24, 2003, p. 2031
19. Bhagat, R. (2002). *"HIV/AIDS in Manipur: In the 'state' of despair."* The Hindu Business Online, July 10, 2002
20. Bharat S, Aggleton P., (1999) *"facing the challenge: household responses to HIV/AIDS in Mumbai, India"*. AIDS Care. 1999 Feb; 11(1):31-44.
21. Boily MC, Lowndes CM, Vickerman P, Kumaranayake L, Blanchard J, Moses S, Ramesh BM, Pickles M, Watts C, Washington R, Reza-Paul S, Labbe AC, Anderson RM, Deering KN, Alary M; (2007) *"CHARME-India team. Evaluating large-scale HIV prevention interventions: study design for an integrated mathematical modeling approach"*. Sexually Transmitted Infection 2007 Dec; 83(7):582-9.
22. Bradley M, Mathers, Louisa Degenhardt, Benjamin Phillips, Lucas Wiessing, Prof Matthew Hickman, Steffanie A Strathdee, Alex Wodak, Samiran Panda, Mark Tyndall, Abdalla Toufik, Richard P Mattick., (2008) *"Reference Group to the UN on HIV and Injecting Drug Use. Global epidemiology of injecting drug use and HIV among people who inject drugs: a systematic review"* The Lancet, Volume 372, Issue 9651, Pages 1733 - 1745, 15 November 2008
23. Budhachandra Y, Ramesh K, Sumitra G., (2007) *"Personality profile among Human Immunodeficiency Virus (HIV) positives and Acquired Immunodeficiency Syndrome (AIDS) patients of injecting drug users"*. Kathmandu

University Medical Journal (KUMJ) 2007 Jan-Mar; 5(1):38-41.

24. Cambodia National AIDS Authority *"The National Strategic Plan for Comprehensive & Multi-Sectoral Response to HIV/ AIDS III (2011-2015) in Cambodia"*
25. Carael M, Marais H, Polsky J, Mendoza A., (2009) *"Is there a gender gap in the HIV response? Evaluating national HIV responses from the United Nations General Assembly Special Session on HIV/AIDS country reports"*. Journal of Acquired Immune Deficiency Syndrome 2009 Dec; 52 Suppl 2:S111-8.
26. Chakrabati S, Panda S, Chatterji A(2000). "*HIV-1 Subtype in Injecting Drug Users to their non Injecting Wives in Manipur, India"*. Indian Journal of Medical Research (III), 189-194, June 2000
27. Charon, (1986), *"Sociology: A Conceptual Approach"*. Boston: Allyn and Bacon. (1986:110, 142)
28. Chawng, Lungmuana., (1999) Impact of Needle Syringe Exchange Programme (NSEP) in One North-Eastern State of India. *The Abstract book of 7th ICAAP Kobe Conference. 1999*
29. Chhabra R, Springer C, Rapkin B, Merchant Y., (2008) *"Differences among male/female adolescents participating in a School-based Teenage Education Program (STEP) focusing on HIV prevention in India"*. Ethnicity & Disesae. 2008 Spring;18(2 Suppl 2):S2-123-7.
30. Cicely Marston, Eleanor King., (2006) *"Factors that shape young people's sexual behaviour: a systematic review"*. The Lancet, Volume 368, Issue 9547, Pages 1581 - 1586, 4 November 2006
31. Commission on AIDS in Asia, (2008). *"Redefining AIDS in Asia: crafting an effective response"*. New Delhi, Oxford University Press.
32. *Constitution for AIDS*. Indian Medical Tribunal 1996 Jan 15; 4(1):3-4.

33. Cornman DH, Schmiege SJ, Bryan A, Benziger TJ, Fisher JD., (2007) *"An information-motivation-behavioral skills (IMB) model-based HIV prevention intervention for truck drivers in India"*. Social Science & Medicine. 2007 Apr; 64(8):1572-84.

34. Crepaz et al, "*Highly active antiretroviral therapy and sexual risk behavior: a meta-analytic review*", JAMA 292(2), 14 July 2004

35. Dandona L, Kumar SG, Kumar GA, Dandona R., (2009) "*Economic analysis of HIV prevention interventions in Andhra Pradesh state of India to inform resource allocation*". AIDS 2009 Jan 14; 23(2):233-42.

36. Dandona L, Kumar SG, Kumar GA, Dandona R., (2009) "*Economic analysis of HIV prevention interventions in Andhra Pradesh state of India to inform resource allocation*". AIDS 2009 Jan 14; 23(2):233-42.

37. Das L. D.K, (2005) "*Designs of Social research"*. Rawat publication, New Delhi

38. De Souza R., (2009) *"Creating communicative spaces: a case of NGO community organizing for HIV and AIDS prevention"*. Health Communication 2009 Dec; 24(8):692-702. Department of Communication, University of Minnesota, Duluth, MN 55812, USA.

39. Deacon, T., (1997) *"The Symbolic Species: The Co-Evolution of Language and the Brain"*. W.W. Norton, New York, p. 25, 1997

40. Deblonde J, De Koker P, Hamers FF, Fontaine J, Luchters S, Temmerman M., (2010) *"Barriers to HIV testing in Europe: a systematic review"*. European Journal of Public Health. 2010 Feb 1.

41. Delva W, Michielsen K, Meulders B, Groeninck S, Wasonga E, Ajwang P, Temmerman M, Vanreusel B., (2010) *"HIV prevention through sport: the case of the Mathare Youth Sport Association in Kenya*". AIDS Care. 2010 Jun 14:1-9. International Centre for Reproductive Health, Faculty of

Medicine and Health Sciences, Ghent University, Ghent, Belgium

42. Dr Athena P Kourtis MD, Francis K Lee PhD, Prof Elaine J Abrams MD, Denise J Jamieson MD, Marc Bulterys MD Nov (2006): *"Mother-to-child transmission of HIV-1: timing and implications for prevention"*. The Lancet Infectious Diseases, Vol. 6 No. 11 pp 726-732
43. Eicher AD, Crofts N, Benjamin S, Deutschmann P, Rodger AJ (2000). *"A certain fate: spread of HIV among young injecting drug users in Manipur, North-East India."* AIDS CARE, Vol. 12, No. 4, pp. 497-504
44. Epidemic of abuse: police harassment of HIV/AIDS outreach workers in India. Human Rights Watch 2002; 14(5) (www.hrw.org/reports/2002/india2/ india0602.pdf). Accessed on 12/7/2014
45. EUROPEAN COMMISSION *"Action Plan on HIV/AIDS in the EU and neighbouring countries: 2014-2016"* Brussels, 14.3.2014 SWD (2014) 106 final
46. F. Ogolla, J. Okungu, V. Kutai, S. Olang'o, S. Wangila, N. Otwoma, M. Ndirangu., (2008) Assessment of client satisfaction on capacity building and grant-making initiatives: the case of AMREF Maanisha Project in Kenya *AIDS 2008 XVII International AIDS Conference Abstracts book 2 pp 294 • 3-8 August 2008, Mexico City*
47. F.C. Iskandar, N. France, F. Wong Commission on AIDS in Asia: genuine community consultation influencing regional recommendations AIDS 2008 *XVII International AIDS Conference Abstracts book 1 pp 264 • 3-8 August 2008, Mexico City*
48. Fakolade R, Adebayo SB, Anyanti J, Ankomah A., (2010) *"the impact of exposure to mass media campaigns and social support on levels and trends of HIV-related stigma and discrimination in Nigeria: tools for enhancing effective HIV prevention programmes"*. Journal Biosocial Science. 2010 May; 42(3):395-407.

49. Farill, E., M. Romero, G. Ornelas, and M. Urbina. (1992) Sex education for priests. *Abstract PoD 5292 at the VIIIth International AIDS Conference, Amsterdam, 19–24 July.*

50. Gammelgaard, J. (1992). *Shifts in drug-taking threaten Asia. World AIDS, No. 21, pp. 5-6. GNP+ (2009, April), 'Living 2008: The Positive Leadership Summit Report'.*

51. *Genesis 1:26-27 The Holy Bible*

52. Global Report 2013, *UNAIDS report on Global AIDS epidemic*

53. GOI, Ministry of Health and Family Welfare, NACO, (2000) Combating HIV/AIDS in India, 2000-2001. Accessed on 1/8/2014

54. GOI, Ministry of health and Family Welfare, National Aids Control Organisation (NACO, 2015) *National AIDS Prevention and Control Policy*

55. Gold, R.S (2006) *"Unrealistic optimism about becoming infected with HIV: Different causes in different population"*. International journal of STD & AIDS, 2006 (mar), vol 17(3), 196-199.

56. Gracious Thomas (2001) *"HIV Education and prevention, looking beyond the present"*. Shipra publication Delhi.

57. Grosso A, Ryan O, Tram KH, Baral S., (2015) *"Financing the response to HIV among gay men and other men who have sex with men: Case studies from eight diverse countries"*. Global Public Health. 2015 Jul 3:1-13.

58. Gruskin S, Ferguson L (2009) *"Government regulation of sex and sexuality: in their own words"*. Reproductive Health Matters. Nov; 17(34):108-18.

59. Gruskin S, Ferguson L (2009) *"Government regulation of sex and sexuality: in their own words"*. Reproductive Health Matters. Nov; 17(34):108-18.

60. Hangzo C, Chatterjee A, Sarkar S, Zomi GT, Deb BC, Abdul-Quader AS *"Reaching out beyond the hills: HIV prevention among injecting drug users in Manipur, India."* Addiction, Vol. 92, No. 7, pp. 813-20

61. Hazarika, Sanjoy (1994) *Strangers of the mist. Tales of War and Peace form India's Northeast,* New Delhi.
62. Hazarika, Sanjoy (1994) *Strangers of the mist. Tales of War and Peace form India's Northeast,* New Delhi.
63. Hazarika, Sanjoy (2000) *The Rites of passage: Border Crossings, Imagined Homelands, India's east and Bangladesh* (Penguin).
64. Hazarika, Sanjoy (2000) *The Rites of passage: Border Crossings, Imagined Homelands, India's east and Bangladesh* (Penguin).
65. Heng Sophea b, Vonthanak Saphonna, Chhorvann Chheaa and Knut Fylkesnes (2009). *"Distribution of HIV in Cambodia: findings from the first national population survey*". AIDS, 23(11):1389–1395.
66. HIV/AIDS and the drug trade Mirante, E. (1993*). "Drug Injecting in Manipur, India. The Burma Connection."* AIDS & Society, Vol. 4, No. 2, p. 4.
67. HIV/AIDS in India. *Report of the Working Group on Global HIV/AIDS and STI Surveillance,* UNAIDS/WHO, Geneva
68. Hogle, Janice, ed. (2002) *"What happened in Uganda? Declining HIV Prevalence, Behavior Change, and the National Response".* Washington, D.C.: U.S. Agency for International Development.
69. Hong Kong Advisory Council on AIDS (Secretariat) *"Recommended HIV/AIDS Strategies for Hong Kong 2012-2016, on firmer ground, strengthening the Hong Kong Response"* 3/F, Wang Tau Hom Jockey Club Clinic, 200 Junction Road East, Kowloon, Hong Kong
70. HRW World Report (2001*) AIDS and Human Rights: A Call for Action,* (June 26).
71. HRW World Report (2001*) AIDS and Human Rights: A Call for Action,* (June 26).
72. HRW World Report (2001) *UN: AIDS Conference Whitewash, US, Vatican, Egypt Undermining frank Language in Conference Document,* (New York, June 20).

73. HRW World Report (2001) *UN: AIDS Conference Whitewash, US, Vatican, Egypt Undermining frank Language in Conference Document,* (New York, June 20).

74. http://www. NACO website, 'About NACO, National AIDS Control Programme Phase 1 (1992-1999)', accessed 4/7/14

75. Human Rights Watch (2002) *"Epidemic of Abuse: police Harassment of HIV/AIDS Outreach Workers in India*", Vol. 14, No. 5 (C)

76. Human Rights Watch (2002) *"Epidemic of Abuse: police Harassment of HIV/AIDS Outreach Workers in India*", Vol. 14, No. 5 (C)

77. Human Science Research Council, (2004) *"an audit of HIV/AIDS policies In Botswana, Lesotho, Mozambique, South Africa, Swaziland and Zimbabwe".* Edited by Nompumelelo Zungu-Dirwayi, M.A., Olive Shisana, Sc.D, Eric Udjo, Ph.D, Thabang Mosala, Ph.D & John Seager, Ph.D

78. Huntington, Dale (2001) "*Anti-Trafficking Programs in South Asia: Appropriate Activities, Indicators and Evaluation Methodologies; Summary Report of a Technical Consultative Meeting"* (Population Council, New Delhi).

79. Huntington, Dale (2001) "*Anti-Trafficking Programs in South Asia: Appropriate Activities, Indicators and Evaluation Methodologies; Summary Report of a Technical Consultative Meeting"* (Population Council, New Delhi)

80. International Crisis Group (2001) "*HIV/AIDS as a Security Issue*" Washington/Brussels)

81. International Crisis Group (2001) "*HIV/AIDS as a Security Issue*" Washington/Brussels)

82. International HIV/AIDS Alliance, *"Positive Prevention: Prevention Strategies for People with HIV/AIDS",* July 2003

83. Iwere, N., J.C. Ojidoh, and N. Okide., (2000) Engaging religious communities in breaking the silence on HIV and AIDS. *Abstract MoPeD2729 at the XIIIth International AIDS Conference, Durban, South Africa, 9–14 July.*

84. Jain, Kalpana (2002) *"Positive Lives: The Story of Ashok and others with HIV"* (Penguin, New Delhi)

85. Jain, Kalpana (2002) *"Positive Lives: The Story of Ashok and others with HIV"* (Penguin, New Delhi)

86. Jaiswal AK, Banerjee S, Grover S.,(2002) *"Changing trends in sexually transmitted diseases in north eastern India"*. Indian Journal of Dermatology, Veneology and leprology, 68(2), 65-66, 2002.

87. Jayasuriya, D. C. (2001) *Background Paper on HIV/AIDS Related National Policies in Selected South and Southwest Asian Countries*

88. Jayasuriya, D. C. (2001) *Background Paper on HIV/AIDS Related National Policies in Selected South and Southwest Asian Countries*

89. John Pickrell (2006) *"Timeline: HIV & AIDS"*, New Scientist, Sept. 4

90. Joseph S, Kielmann K, Kudale A, Sheikh K, Shinde S, Porter J, Rangan S.,(2010) *"Examining sex differentials in the uptake and process of HIV testing in three high prevalence districts of India"*. AIDS Care. 2010 Mar; 22(3):286-95.

91. Kagimu, M., E. Marum, F. Wabwire-Mangen, N. Nakyanjo, Y. Walakira, and J. Hogle., (1998) *"Evaluation of the effectiveness of AIDS health education interventions in the Muslim community in Uganda"*. AIDS Education Prevention 10(3):215–228.

92. Kaleeba, N., J. Namulondo, D. Kalinki, and G. Williams., (2000) *"Open secret: People facing up to HIV and AIDS in Uganda"*. Strategies for Hope Series No. 15. London: ActionAid.

93. Kalichman S. (ed) (2006), *"Positive Prevention: Reducing HIV Transmission Among People Living with HIV/AIDS"* Springer.

94. Kaye Wellings, Martine Collumbien, Emma Slaymaker, Susheela Singh, Zoé Hodges, Dhaval Patel., (2006): *"HIV prevention, treatment, and care services for people who*

inject drugs: a systematic review of global, regional, and national coverage". The Lancet, Vol. 368 No. 9548 pp 1706-1728

95. Kennedy et al,(2007) "The impact of HIV treatment on risk behavour in developing countries: A systematic review", AIDS Care 19(6), July 2007
96. Kennedy.,(2007) *"The impact of HIV treatment on risk behavour in developing countries: A systematic review"*, AIDS Care 19(6), July 2007
97. Khan, M. Z., (1985) "*Drug use amongst the college youth*" Somaiya publications, New Delhi.
98. Kheirandish P, Seyedalinaghi SA, Hosseini M, Jahani MR, Shirzad H, Foroughi M, Ahmadian MR, Jabbari H, Mohraz M, McFarland W., (2010) *"Prevalence and correlates of HIV infection among male injection drug users in detention in Tehran, Iran"*. Journal of Acquired Immune Deficiency Syndrome. 2010 Feb 1; 53(2):273-5
99. Lal P, Singh MM, Malhotra R, Ingle GK.,(2007) *"Perception of risk and potential occupational exposure to HIV/AIDS among medical interns in Delhi"*. Journal of Communicable Disease 2007 Jun; 39(2):95-9.
100. Lamptey and Price,(1998) "*Social marketing sexually transmitted disease and HIV prevention: a consumer-centered approach to achieving behavior change*", AIDS 12 Suppl 2, 1998
101. Lamptey and Price., (1998) *"Social marketing sexually transmitted disease and HIV prevention: a consumer-centered approach to achieving behavior change"*, AIDS 12 Suppl 2, 1998
102. Lazzarini, Z. (1998) *Human rights and HIV and AIDS. Discussion Papers on HIV AND AIDS Care and Support. Paper No. 2. Washington, D.C.: USAID/The Synergy Project.*
103. Lee, Tony Szu-Hsien; Fu, Li-An, Fleming Paul., (2006) *"Using focus group to investigate the educational needs of female injecting Heroin users in Taiwan in relation to*

HIV/AIDS prevention". Health education research, 2006 (feb), vol 21(1), 55-65.

104. Li L, Rotheram-Borus MJ, Lu Y, Wu Z, Lin C, Guan J., (2009) *"Mass media and HIV and AIDS in China"*. Journal of Health Communication. 2009 Jul-Aug; 14(5):424-38. Semel Institute for Neuroscience and Human Behavior, Center for Community Health, University of California at Los Angeles, Los Angeles, California 90024, USA.

105. Lisam D.R., (2002) Translating Knowledge and experience into policy change and action success stories from Manipur, India. *Book of XVI International AIDS Conference, Barcelona, July 2002*

106. M. Shanmugam, K. Govindaswamy, P. Babu, S. Balasubramania, S. Varadhan, S.S. Goh Community-specific advocacy action plan to promote health/rights of vulnerable communities and PLHIV networks in Tamil Nadu, India *AIDS 2008 XVII International AIDS Conference Abstracts book 1 pp 264 -3-8 August 2008, Mexico City*

107. Malhotra R, Malhotra C, Sharma N., (2008) *"should there be mandatory testing for HIV prior to marriage in India"?* Indian Journal of Medical Ethics. 2008 Apr-Jun; 5(2):70-4.

108. Marston and King, *"Factors that shape young people's sexual behaviour: a systematic review"*, Lancet 368(9547), 4 November 2006

109. Marston and King,(2006) *"Factors that shape young people's sexual behaviour: a systematic review"*, Lancet 368(9547), 4 November 2006

110. Mathew, P.D (1996) "*AIDS and Law*". Indian Social Institute, New Delhi.

111. Maticka-Tyndale E, Barnett JP, (2010) *"Peer-led interventions to reduce HIV risk of youth: a review"*. Evaluation Program Planning. 2010 May; 33(2):98-112.

112. Mayer K. & Pizer H. (eds) (2009), *'HIV Prevention: A Comprehensive Approach'*.

113. Michael P, Johnson 1999 *"Personal, Moral and Structural Commitment to Relationship experiences of choices and constraints"* Springer US ISBN 978-1-4613-7161-8 pp 73-87

114. Michael P, Johnson 1999 *"Personal, Moral and Structural Commitment to Relationship experiences of choices and constraints"* Springer US ISBN 978-1-4613-7161-8 pp 73-87

115. Ministry of Health, State Development Planning Commission *"China's National Medium-and Long-Term Strategic Plan for HIV/AIDS Prevention and Control (1998-2010)"*

116. Mittal D, Babitha GA, Prakash S, Kumar N, Prashant GM. (2015).,"*Knowledge and Attitude about HIV/AIDS among HIV-Positive Individuals in Davangere*". Social Work in Public Health 2015 Aug-Sep; 30(5):423-30.

117. NACO (2006). *HIV/AIDS in India an update*

118. NACO (April 2006), *HIV/AIDS epidemiological Surveillance & Estimation report for the year 2005*

119. NACO, *HIV Sentinel Surveillance 2013 India Country Report*

120. National AIDS Control Organisation (2012). *UNGASS country progress report 2013: India. New Delhi, Ministry of Health and Family Welfare.*

121. National AIDS Control Organisation, National Institute of Health & Family Welfare (2012). *Annual HIV sentinel surveillance: country report, 2013. New Delhi, National Institute of Health and Family Welfare, National AIDS Control Organisation.*

122. National HIV/AIDS Policy Jamaica 2005

123. National HIV/AIDS Strategy (NHAS) of United States of America July 2010

124. Newman PA, Rubincam C, Slack C, Essack Z, Chakrapani V, Chuang DM, Tepjan S, Shunmugam M, Roungprakhon S, Logie C, Koen J, Lindegger G.2015 *"Towards a Science*

of Community Stakeholder Engagement in Biomedical HIV Prevention Trials: An Embedded Four-Country Case Study". PLoS One. 2015 Aug 21;10(8)

125. Nitsoy, R. Zaika., (2008) Policy implications of national AIDS spending assessment in Ukraine *AIDS 2008 XVII International AIDS Conference Abstracts pp 263 • 3-8 August 2008, Mexico City*

126. Nyamathi A, Thomas B, Greengold B, Swaminathan S., (2009) "*Perceptions and health care needs of HIV-Positive mothers in India*". Programme on Community Health and Partnership 2009 summer; 3(2):99-108.

127. Ojha V, P, B (2006). *The Macro-Economic and Sectoral Impacts of HIV and AIDS in India, UNDP,NCAER,NACO 2006*

128. Panda S (1994). *"Epidemic of Herpes Zoster following HIV epidemics in Manipur, India"*. Journal of Infections 128(2), 167-173, March 1994

129. Panda S et al (2000) "*Transmission of HIV from injection drug users to their wives in India*". International Journal of STD and AIDS 2000, 11: 468-473

130. Panda S, Bijaya L, Sadhana Devi N, Foley E, Chatterjee A, Banerjee D, Naik TN, Saha MK, Bhattacharya SK (2001). *"Interface between drug use and sex work in Manipur."* The National Medical Journal of India, Vol. 14, No. 4, pp. 209-1

131. Panda S, Bijaya L, Sadhana Devi N, Foley E, Chatterjee A, Banerjee D, Naik TN, Saha MK, Bhattacharya SK (2001). *"Interface between drug use and sex work in Manipur."* The National Medical Journal of India, Vol. 14, No. 4, pp. 209-11

132. Panda S, Chatterjee A, Bhattacharya SK, Manna B, Singh PN, Sarkar S, Naik TN, Chakrabarti S, Detels R (2000). *"Transmission of HIV from injecting drug users to their wives in India."* International Journal of STD & AIDS, Vol. 11, pp. 468-73

133. Patterson, Brent and Francis Robichaud,(1996) *"Managing your Health, a guide for people living with HIV or AIDS"*, CATIE, RCITS, and TPWAF, 1996.

134. Paul Arora, Rajesh Kumar, Madhulekha Bhattacharya, Nico JD Nagelkerke , Prabhat Jha (2008). *"Trends in HIV incidence in India from 2000 to 2007"*. Lancet, 372(9635):289–290.

135. Peersman and Levy, *"Focus and effectiveness of HIV-prevention efforts for young people"*, AIDS 12 Suppl A, 1998

136. Peersman G, Ferguson L, Torres MA, Smith S, Gruskin S., (2009) *"Increasing civil society participation in the national HIV response: the role of UNGASS reporting"* Journal of Acquired Immune Deficiency Syndrome 2009 Dec; 52 Suppl 2:S97-103.

137. Pisal H, Sutar S, Sastry J, Kapadia-Kundu N, Joshi A, Joshi M, Leslie J, Scotti L, Bharucha K, Suryavanshi N, Phadke M, Bollinger R, Shankar AV., (2007) *"Nurses' health education program in India increases HIV knowledge and reduces fear"*. Journal of Association of Nurses and AIDS Care. 2007 Nov-Dec; 18(6):32-43.

138. Punde PA, Punde S., (2014) *"Comprehensive Survey to Study Awareness, Knowledge and Attitude towards HIV/AIDS and Hepatitis B amongst Dental Professionals Working in Rural India"*. Journal Maxillofacial and Oral Surgery. 2014 Dec; 13(4):483-7.

139. Rafiey H, Narenjiha H, Shirinbayan P, Noori R, Javadipour M, Roshanpajouh M, Samiei M, Assari S., (2009) *"Needle and syringe sharing among Iranian drug injectors"*. Harm Reduction Journal. 2009 Jul 30; 6:21

140. Ramdurg S, Ambekar A, Lal R., (2015) *"Co-relationship between sexual dysfunction and high-risk sexual behavior in patients receiving buprenorphine and naltrexone maintenance therapy for opioid dependence"*. Industrial Psychiatry Journal. 2015 Jan-Jun; 24(1):29-34.

141. Ramesh, Banadakoppa M; Moses, Stephen; Washington, Reynold; Isac, Shajy; Mohapatra, Bidhubhushan; Mahagaonkar, Sangameshwar B; Adhikary, Rajatashuvra; Brahmam, Ginnela NV; Paranjape, Ramesh S; Subramanian, Thilakavathi; Blanchard, James F; for the IBBA Study Team (2008). "*Determinants of HIV prevalence among female sex workers in four south Indian states: analysis of cross-sectional surveys in twenty-three districts*". AIDS, 22 (Supp. 5):S35–S44.

142. Ramiah, I (July, 2004). Securitizing the HIV/AIDS Issue in Asia

143. Richardson et al, "*Effect of brief safer-sex counseling by medical providers to HIV-1 seropositive patients: a multi-clinic assessment*", AIDS 18(8), May 2004

144. Riehman, K.S. (1996). "*Injecting Drug Use and AIDS in Developing Countries: Determinants and Issues for Policy Consideration.*" Paper prepared for the Policy Research Report on AIDS and Development,World Bank, Policy Research Department, October

145. Roger AJ, Tode M, Lalnunthiangi B, Muan V. DOTS based Tuberculosis treatment and control during civil conflict and an HIV epidemic in Churachandpur District, India. Bulletin of the World Health Organisation 180(6) 451-456, 2002.

146. Romer D, Sznitman S, DiClemente R, Salazar LF, Vanable PA, Carey MP, Hennessy M, Brown LK, Valois RF, Stanton BF, Fortune T, Juzang I., (2009) "*Mass media as an HIV-prevention strategy: using culturally sensitive messages to reduce HIV-associated sexual behavior of at-risk African American youth*". American Journal of Public Health. 2009 Dec; 99(12):2150-9.

147. Rupani MP, Pawar AB, Bansal RK, Patel PB, Shah PS, Parikh KD,. 2015 "*Cross-sectional study on socio-demographic and clinical correlates of depression among human immunodeficiency virus-positive patients in Surat City, Western India*". Asia Pacific Psychiatry. 2015 Jun 24.

148. S. Bhagyabati Devi, Singh T.J. Naorem S., (2005) *"HIV and TB Co-infection: A study from RIMS Hospital, Manipur"* Journal of Indian Academy of clinical Medicine, 6(3), 220-223, July, Sept. 2005

149. S. Bhagyabati Devi, Singh TJ., (2003) *"Recent trend of TB, a possible impact of HIV infection: a study in Regional Institute of Medical Sciences Hospital, Imphal"*. JAPI 2003

150. S. Gruskin., (2002) *"The UN General Assembly Special Session on HIV/AIDS: were some lessons of the last 20 years ignored."?* American Journal of Public Health 2002; 92(3): 337-338.

151. S.L Goel and R. Kumar (2004), *"Administration and management of NGO's"* Deep and Deep Publications pvt. Ltd. New Delhi.

152. Sachdev P., (1998) *"AIDS/HIV and university students in Delhi, India: knowledge, beliefs, attitudes and behaviors".* School of Social Work, Indiana University, Indianapolis 46202, USA. Social Work Health Care. 1998; 26(4):37-57.

153. Samuel Siringi, March (2010) *"HIV/AIDS on the rise in young people in Kenya"* The Lancet Infectious Diseases, Volume 10, Issue 3, Page 149, March 2010

154. Sarin E, Selhore E., (2008) *"Serving women who use drugs in Delhi, India: challenges and achievements".* International Journal on Drug Policy 2008 Apr; 19(2):176-8

155. Sarkar K, Panda S, Das N, Sarkar S (1997). *"Relationship of National Highway with injecting drug abuse and HIV in rural Manipur, India."* Indian Journal of Public Health, Vol. 41, No. 2, pp. 49-51.

156. Sarkar NN., (2008) *"Barriers to condom use"*. European Journal of Contraceptive and Reproductive Health Care. 2008 Jun; 13(2):114-22. Department of Reproductive Biology, All India Institute of Medical Sciences, New Delhi, India.

157. Sarkar S, Das N, Panda S, Naik TN, Sarkar K, Singh BC, Ralte JM, Aier SM, Tripathy SP (1993). *"Rapid spread of HIV among injecting drug-users in north-eastern states of*

India." Bulletin on Narcotics, Vol. 45, No. 1, pp. 91-105

158. Sarkar S, Panda S, Sarkar K, Hangzo CZ, Bijaya L, Singh NY, Das N, Agarwal A, Chatterjee A (1995). *"A cross-sectional study on factors including HIV testing and counseling determining unsafe injecting practices among injecting drug users of Manipur."* Indian Journal of Public Health, Vol. 39, No. 3, pp. 86-92.

159. Sastry S., (2015) "*Long Distance Truck Drivers and the Structural Context of Health: A Culture-Centered Investigation of Indian Truckers' Health Narratives*". Health Communication. 2015 Aug 12:1-12.

160. Sayeda Urooj (2006) "*Community participation in the targeted interventions programme for HIV/AIDS prevention: A Study of NGOs in Delhi*". M.Phil Thesis, Department of Social Work, University of Delhi.

161. Seloilwe, Esther S (2005) *"factors that influence the spread of HIV/AIDS among student of the university of Botswana"* JANAC journal of the association of nurses in AIDS care 2005 may – june vol 16 (3),3-10.

162. Singh B, Ngangom S. (8-12 Nov. 1992) Abstract book of the 2nd International Congress on AIDS in ASIA and the pacific Ashok Hotel New Delhi

163. Singh H, Dulhani N, Bithika NK, Tiwari P, Chauhan V, Singh P., (2010) *"Rural Epidemiology of HIV Positive Tribal Patients from Chhattisgarh in India"*. Journal of Global Infectious Disease. 2010 Jan; 2(1):39-42.

164. Singh IP., (1998) "*STD-HIV intervention programme: the Sonagachi model*" Health Millions 1998 Jan-Feb; 24(1):11-3.

165. Singh NB, Brojachand (1993) *"Drug related HIV infection/ AIDS in Manipur and the North Eastern states of India"*. Journal ISHA-1993

166. Singh O.H. (August 2006). A month long drug use and HIV/AIDS campaign in Imphal city. *Abstract book of XVI International AIDS Conference, Toronto, Social Action and Service Organisation*

167. Singh TN, Kananbala S, Thongam W, Devi KhS, Singh NB (2005). *"Increasing trend of HIV seropositivity among commercial sex workers attending the Voluntary and Confidential Counseling and Testing Centre in Manipur, India."* International Journal of STD & AIDS, Vol. 16: 166–169

168. Singhall, A and Rogers, E M (2003), *"Combating AIDS: communication strategies in action"* London: SAGE

169. Sivaram S, Zelaya C, Srikrishnan AK, Latkin C, Go VF, Solomon S, Celentano D. (2009) *"Associations between social capital and HIV stigma in Chennai, India: considerations for prevention intervention design"*. AIDS Education Preview 2009 Jun; 21(3):233-50

170. Sopheab H, Saphonna V., Chheaa C., Fylkesnes K., (2009) *"Distribution of HIV in Cambodia: findings from the first national population survey"*. AIDS 2009, 23:1389–1395

171. South African National AIDS Council (SANAC) *"National Strategic Plan on HIV, STIs and TB 2012-2016"*

172. Subramanian, K.S (2002). *Impact of conflict on HIV/AIDS in south Asia*

173. Sue Perry., (2002) *southern Africa regional co-ordination world council of churches, ecumenical HIV and AIDS initiatives in Africa (EHAIA).*

174. T Azim , M Rahman , M S Alam , I A Chowdhury, R Khan, M Reza, M Rahman, E I Chowdhury MSS *, M Hanifuddin MBBS MPH and A S M M Rahman FRCP (2008). *"Bangladesh moves from being a low-prevalence nation for HIV to one with a concentrated epidemic in injecting drug users*". International Journal of STD & AIDS, 19:327–331,

175. Takei T , Amin NA, Schmid G, Dhingra-Kumar N, Rugg D. (2009), *"Progress in Global Blood Safety for HIV"* Journal of Acquired Immune Deficiency Syndromes 52.

176. Tarun Bikash Sukai (2010) "*AIDS NGO's and Globalisation*" Akansha Publishing house, New Delhi. pp171-239

177. *Thailand National AIDS Strategy 2012-16*
178. The European Mode of Delivery Collaboration, *"Elective caesarean-section versus vaginal delivery in prevention of vertical HIV-1 transmission: a randomised clinical trial",* The Lancet 353(9165), March 1999
179. The International Perinatal HIV Group, *"The mode of delivery and the risk of vertical transmission of human immunodeficiency virus type 1—a meta-analysis of 15 prospective cohort studies",* NEJM 340(13), April 1999
180. *The National HIV Prevention Action Plan Volume 3: June 2011 Kampala, Uganda*
181. Thomas B, Nyamathi A, Swaminathan S., (2009) *"Impact of HIV/AIDS on mothers in southern India: a qualitative study"*.AIDS and Behaviour Oct; 13(5):989-96
182. Thomas B, Nyamathi A, Swaminathan S.,(2009) *"Impact of HIV/AIDS on mothers in southern India: a qualitative study"*.AIDS and Behaviour 2009 Oct; 13(5):989-96
183. Thomas B.E, Chandra S, Selvi KJ, Suriyanarayanan D, Swaminathan S., (2009) *"Gender differences in sexual behaviour among people living with HIV in Chennai, India".* Indian Journal of Medical Research 2009 Jun; 129(6):690-4.
184. Thomas J, Bandyopadhyay M., (1999) *"Ethnic minorities and their vulnerability to AIDS in a border state of India".* AIDS Care. 1999 Feb; 11(1):45-60.
185. Thomas, J. and M. Bandyopadhyay (1999). *"Ethnic Minorities and their vulnerability to AIDS in a border state of India."* AIDS CARE, Vol. 11, No. 1, pp. 45-60
186. Ucheaga DN, Hartwig KA., *"2010 Religious leaders' response to AIDS in Nigeria".* Glob Public Health. 2010 Feb 10:1-15
187. UNAIDS (*1997) "Blood safety and HIV",*
188. UNAIDS (2005) *From advocacy to action: a progress report on UNAIDS at country level*

189. UNAIDS (2007) *"Practical Guidelines for Intensifying HIV Prevention"*

190. UNAIDS (2012) *"Regional HIV and AIDS statistics"*

191. UNAIDS (Joint United Nations Program on HIV/AIDS) / WHO (World Health Organization), 2002.

192. UNAIDS (Joint United Nations Program on HIV/AIDS), 1998a. *AIDS and the Military, A UNAIDS Point of View.* UNAIDS, Geneva.

193. UNAIDS (Joint United Nations Program on HIV/AIDS), 1998b. *AIDS Education through Imams.* UNAIDS, Geneva.

194. UNAIDS (Joint United Nations Program on HIV/AIDS), 1999. *From Principle to Practice, Greater Involvement of People Living with or Affected by HIV/AIDS.* UNAIDS, Geneva.

195. UNAIDS (Joint United Nations Program on HIV/AIDS), 2001. *Population, Mobility and AIDS.* UNAIDS Technical Update. UNAIDS, Geneva.

196. UNAIDS (Joint United Nations Program on HIV/AIDS), 2002. *HIV/AIDS in Asia.* UNAIDS, Geneva.

197. UNAIDS (Joint United Nations Program on HIV/AIDS), 2002. *Human Resources and Sustainable Development, an Overview Report on HIV's Impacts on Human Resources.* UNAIDS, Geneva.

198. UNAIDS (Joint United Nations Program on HIV/AIDS), 2003a. *AIDS Epidemic Update 2013.* UNAIDS, Geneva.

199. UNAIDS (Joint United Nations Program on HIV/AIDS), 2003b. *On the front line, a review of Policies and Programs to Address HIV/AIDS among peacekeepers and uniformed services.* UNAIDS, Geneva.

200. UNAIDS (Joint United Nations Program on HIV/AIDS), 2003c. *Co-ordination of National Responses to HIV/AIDS, Guiding Principles for National Authorities and their Partners.* UNAIDS, Geneva.

201. UNAIDS (Joint United Nations Program on HIV/AIDS), IPS (Institute of Policy Studies)/ PAHO/, 2001. *NGOs the*

driving force behind public Policy on AIDS. Accessed on Jan 20, 2013 from http://www.ipsnews.net/aids/page_7.shtml

202. UNAIDS *epidemic updates 2013*
203. UNAIDS, *"Sexual behavoural change for HIV: Where have theories taken us?", 1999*
204. UNAIDS, *"The impact of Voluntary Counselling and Testing", 2001*
205. Van Dam C.J., (1994) *"Sexually transmitted diseases and HIV infection: implications for control and prevention"*. Journal of Indian Medical Association 1994 Jan; 92(1):8-10.
206. Van Rompay KK, Madhivanan P, Rafiq M, Krupp K, Chakrapani V, Selvam D., (2008) *"Empowering the people: Development of an HIV peer education model for low literacy rural communities in India"*. Human Resource and Health. 2008 Apr 18; 6:6.
207. Vejella S, Patel SK, Saggurti N, Prabhakar P.(2015) *"Community Collectivization and Consistent Condom Use Among Female Sex Workers in Southern India: Evidence from Two Rounds of Behavioral Tracking Surveys"*. AIDS and Behaviour. 2015 Aug 19.
208. Verma R, Khanna P, Chawla S, Dhankar M.2015 *"HIV vaccine: Can it develop in the 21st century"?*. Human Vaccine & Immunotherapeutic. 2015 Jul 25:0.
209. Vijay P. Ojha and Basanta K. Pradhan 2006 *"The Macro-Economic and Sectoral Impacts of HIV and AIDS in India, A CGE Analysis"* UNDP, NVAER, NACO
210. Wang, Lu; Wang, Ning; Wang, Liyan; Li, Dongmin; Jia, Manhong; Gao, Xing; Qu, Shuquan; Qin, Qianqian; Wang, Yanhe; Smith, Kumi., (2009) *"The 2007 estimates for people at risk for and living with HIV in China: progress and challenges"*. Journal of Acquired Immune Deficiency Syndromes, 50:414–418
211. Wang, Lu; Wang, Ning; Wang, Liyan; Li, Dongmin; Jia, Manhong; Gao, Xing; Qu, Shuquan; Qin, Qianqian; Wang, Yanhe; Smith, Kumi (2009). "The 2007 estimates for people

at risk for and living with HIV in China: progress and challenges". Journal of Acquired Immune Deficiency Syndromes, 50:414–418

212. Weinstein, N. D. (1980) *"Unrealistic optimism about future life events". Journal of Personality and Social Psychology, 39*(5), 806-820.

213. Whiteside Alan, Catarina Andrade, Lisa Arrehag, Solomon Dlamini, Themba Ginindza, Anokhi Parikh (2006). *The socio-economic impact of HIV/AIDS in Swaziland, Durban, South Africa, Health Economics and HIV/AIDS Research Division.*

214. WHO, *"Aide-Memoire for National Blood Programmes",* July 2002

215. WHO, *"Effectiveness of Community-based Outreach in Preventing HIV/AIDS Among Injecting Drug Users",* April 2004

216. WHO, *"Effectiveness of Sterile Needle and Syringe Programming in Reducing HIV/AIDS Among Injecting Drug Users",* January 2005

217. WHO, *"Universal Precautions, Including Injection Safety*

218. Wouters E, van Rensburg HC, Meulemans H., (2010) "*The National Strategic Plan of South Africa: what are the prospects of success after the repeated failure of previous AIDS policy*? Health Policy Plan. 2010 May; 25(3):171-85.

219. Zunyou Wu, Sheena G Sullivan, Yu Wang, Mary Jane Rotheram-Borus, Roger Detels (2007*) "Evolution of China's response to HIV/AIDS*" Lancet 2007; Volume 369: PP 679–90

Index